REA

ACPL ITEM
DISCARDED

How to Use Control Charts for Healthcare

D. Lynn Kelley

JAN 1 7 2006

Also available from Quality Press

Healthcare Performance Measurements: Systems Design and Evaluation
Vahé A. Kazandjian and Terry R. Lied

Stop Managing Costs: Designing Healthcare Organizations around Core Business Systems
James P. Mozena, Charles E. Emerick, and Steven C. Black

Statistical Quality Control Using Excel
Steven M. Zimmerman, Ph.D. and Marjorie L. Icenogle, Ph.D.

The Handbook for Managing Change in Healthcare
ASQ Healthcare Series, Chip Caldwell editor

Statistical Analysis for Decision Makers in Healthcare: Understanding and Evaluating Critical Information in a Competitive Market
Jeffrey C. Bauer

Transforming Health Care: Action Strategies for Health Care Leaders
Daniel J. Anderson, John W. Moran, Baird K. Brightman, and Barry S. Scheur

Using Design Experiments to Shrink Healthcare Costs
M. Daniel Sloan

101 Good Ideas: How to Improve Just About Any Process
Karen Bemowski and Brad Stratton, editors

Quality Problem Solving
Gerald F. Smith

To request a complimentary catalog of ASQ Quality Press publications, call 800-248-1946.

How to Use Control Charts for Healthcare

D. Lynn Kelley

ASQ Quality Press
Milwaukee, Wisconsin

How to Use Control Charts for Healthcare
D. Lynn Kelley

Library of Congress Cataloging-in-Publication Data

Kelley, D. Lynn.
How to use control charts for healthcare / D. Lynn Kelley.
p. cm.
ISBN 0-87389-452-9 (alk. paper)
1. Medical care—Quality control. 2. Quality control—Charts, diagrams, etc. I. Title.
RA399.A1K45 1999
362.1'068'5—dc21 99-31147
CIP

© 1999 by ASQ

All rights reserved. No part of this book may be reproduced in any form or by any means, electronic, mechanical, photocopying, recording, or otherwise, without the prior written permission of the publisher.

10 9 8 7 6 5 4

ISBN 0-87389-452-9

Acquisitions Editor: Ken Zielske
Project Editor: Annemieke Koudstaal
Production Coordinator: Shawn Dohogne

ASQ Mission: The American Society for Quality advances individual and organizational performance excellence worldwide by providing opportunities for learning, quality improvement, and knowledge exchange.

Attention: Bookstores, Wholesalers, Schools, and Corporations:
ASQ Quality Press books, videotapes, audiotapes, and software are available at quantity discounts with bulk purchases for business, educational, or instructional use. For information, please contact ASQ Quality Press at 800-248-1946, or write to ASQ Quality Press, P.O. Box 3005, Milwaukee, WI 53201-3005.

To place orders or to request a free copy of the ASQ Quality Press Publications Catalog, including ASQ membership information, call 800-248-1946. Visit our Web site at http://www.asq.org.

Printed in the United States of America

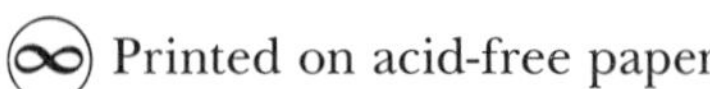

American Society for Quality

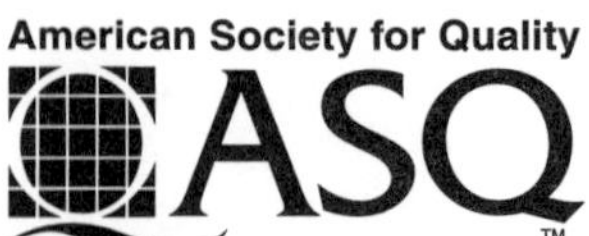

Quality Press
611 East Wisconsin Avenue
Milwaukee, Wisconsin 53202
Call toll free 800-248-1946
http://www.asq.org
http://standardsgroup.asq.org

Table of Contents

3 1833 04968 0827

Acknowledgments

This book is dedicated to Judy Homa-Lowry, as the compelling force behind it. Her insistence that "there is a need for this book" made it a reality. Judy served as the primary advisor to the book. Her insights and advice were invaluable. In addition to reading the book and providing feedback, she wrote several sections, which have been incorporated into the book.

A very special thanks to Greg Gruska who carefully read every word written, spent many hours responding to my e-mail queries, developed several diagrams, wrote actual text, and made numerous suggestions for improving the book.

Early on, Frank Angileri—a quality expert in his own right—spent many hours gathering articles and data for the book. He continued to "feed me" articles throughout the course of writing the book, as well as feeding me "real Italian food" with his wife, Bessie, to nurture my spirits along the way.

Thanks to my husband, Paul, for his love and support. And finally, Krista and Ryan, who provide my life with lots of common cause variation—and that occasional special cause variation that makes parenting what it is.

Preface

The idea for this book was formed after Judy Homa-Lowry and I finished teaching a course called Accreditation Standards for Improving Organization Performance: Using PI Tools and Techniques. The course is sponsored by the Joint Commission on Accreditation of Healthcare Organizations (JCAHO). As we sat down to debrief, we realized we were both amazed at the numerous participant questions regarding control charts. The participants came from many hospitals throughout the country. As much as we tried to bring the focus back to the outlined program, the participants continued to steer the discussion toward control charts.

As we continued to teach around the country (both individually and together), the pattern repeated itself. Many quality professionals in hospitals were excited about control charts. They wanted to use them because they were unhappy with the way they've been analyzing and displaying their data in the past. Some people were so desperate to use control charts that they were performing the calculations by hand or had personally programmed the formulas into spreadsheet packages. Others did not realize that there are many control charts, so they were using the same one over and over for every data set.

Although there are many good books on the market for control charts, there are few that are geared specifically toward healthcare.

There are quite a few books that cover the quality tools for healthcare, but not many of those dedicate much space to control charts. Finally, even the small number of books that do exist on control chart use in healthcare, do not provide the links between control charts and JCAHO requirements. This book is dedicated to the use of control charts in healthcare. The examples that are offered span a wide variety of healthcare applications including (but not limited to) nursing, dietary, finance, and outpatient centers. References to JCAHO requirements are liberally sprinkled throughout the book, including some examples of how to meet many of the JCAHO-required measurements with control charts.

As most healthcare professionals are aware, JCAHO has recently required that organizations differentiate between common and special cause variation. Another JCAHO standard addresses process stability. Both of these standards point firmly in the direction of control chart use—since control charts provide one of the few ways to determine the two types of variation and process stability.

The first chapter of this book gives an introduction to quality and measurement in general (chapter 1), followed by specific steps for introducing quality in healthcare organizations (chapter 2). The information provided in chapter 2 relates specifically to healthcare organizations with JCAHO's accreditation standards in mind. Chapters 3 through 7 provide information on control charts, while the final two chapters show the links between commonly used statistical tools and control charts (chapter 8), and JCAHO's Performance Improvement (PI) standards as they relate to the tools and techniques of quality (chapter 9).

CHAPTER 1

Quality and Measurement in Healthcare

The pressures on healthcare organizations and the healthcare industry in general are tremendous—and appear to be increasing. Patients are demanding better service, litigation is on the rise, third-party payers are paying less and less for services, and regulatory agencies want hospitals to "show compliance." Wouldn't it be nice if there was a *magic spell* that would fix everything? As you know, magic spells are in fairy tales. However, there is hope in quality improvement and its accompanying tools and techniques. Quality improvement is not magic, but the quality philosophy of continuous improvement has helped many organizations meet these increasing challenges and pressures.

What Is Quality?

Quality is known by many names, such as Total Quality Management (TQM), continuous improvement, performance improvement, and process improvement. The Joint Commission on Accreditation of Healthcare Organizations (JCAHO, or Joint Commission) refers to quality as Improving Organizational Performance (IOP), and has a section of standards called the PI (Performance Improvement) standards that relate specifically to the concepts embedded in quality. Although PI is the terminology used by JCAHO, many organizations outside of healthcare use the terminology of QI—or Quality Improvement—to mean essentially the same thing. Throughout this book, the terms Performance Improvement (PI) and Quality Improvement (QI) have been used interchangeably.

Quality has as many definitions as it has names. Several years ago a standard definition was *meeting customer expectations.* That definition was revised to become *exceeding customer expectations.* Some people have referred to quality as the process of *delighting the customer.* Others have said that quality is continuous improvement of organizational products and services. For the purposes of this book, we have defined quality, in a manner similar to JCAHO, as follows:

Quality is continually improving organizational performance.

Now, let's take a look at how continually improving organizational performance can help with the pressures mentioned in the first paragraph.

Patient Demands

A key component of any quality improvement initiative is to obtain feedback from the customer. One of the primary customers in healthcare is the patient. As healthcare organizations begin to gather patient feedback and respond accordingly, patient satisfaction will increase.

Regulatory/Accreditation Agencies

An important requirement of these agencies is to "show them the data." The tools and techniques in quality improvement are data-driven. The tools presented in this book will assist organizations in meeting the requirements of these agencies. In many cases, the links with the Joint Commission requirements are provided in this book. Another characteristic of these agencies is that the *rules* change every few years. Quality tools and techniques help organizations become flexible and nimble to respond to changing environments and regulations.

Overall Pressure to Lower Cost at the Expense of Quality Care

There is a constant pressure on healthcare organizations to lower costs. Management is sometimes so busy tracking costs that they neglect the measurement and improvement of clinical outcomes. Quality initiatives remind us that cost is just one element of providing quality care. The tools in quality improvement help to lower costs and find efficiencies; however, they also help organizations to monitor clinical outcomes and apply continuous improvement to those outcomes.

Litigation

Improving an organization involves improving the quality of care by providing training and development of healthcare employees. When healthcare employees increase their skill levels and become better listeners, the potential for malpractice litigation decreases.

Who Is the Customer in Healthcare?

One of the first considerations in quality improvement is to identify the customer. Most organizations have more than one customer. Think of a customer as someone for whom you provide services, products, or information. Many healthcare organizations separate their customers into two groups: internal and external. *External customers* are those individuals who are outside of the organization. Examples might be the healthcare organization's patients or third-party payers. *Internal customers* are individuals within the organization for whom services are provided. Examples of internal customers in healthcare might be the laboratory department that provides services ordered by an Emergency Room physician. The Emergency Room physician is therefore an internal customer of the laboratory department. In some cases, it is possible for a customer to be both internal and external. For example, a physician may be an internal customer while inside the hospital, and an external customer while working in a private practice.

Overview of Quality Improvement

Quality improvement is not new. It originated in the manufacturing industry many years ago. One major advantage of this situation is that healthcare has the benefit of learning from manufacturing's mistakes. In many cases, we know what works and what doesn't work in quality improvement. For example, in the 1980s, many organizations adopted "quality circles" because of their success in Japan. Today, most U.S. companies have abandoned quality circles because, among other reasons, they were not as effective in the American culture as they were in the Japanese culture. Conversely, many of the tools (such as control charts) have been in use for more than 70 years in the United States. Their effectiveness has been shown in many organizations with multiple applications. Software packages have been developed to support these tools—healthcare doesn't have to start from ground zero.

Most people are familiar with Dr. W. Edwards Deming. Today he is considered one of the preeminent *quality gurus.* In 1950, Deming was invited to speak to Japan's leading industrialists. At that time, Japanese industries were interested in shedding their *shoddy goods* image. Deming's philosophy of quality improvement, paired with the Japanese culture, enabled Japanese industries to rise to world dominance in many areas. Ultimately, U.S. manufacturers adopted Deming's philosophies and tools and were able to regain lost market share. Nationally, the United States has placed such an emphasis on quality that in 1987 it started the Malcolm Baldrige National Quality Award. The award was designed to promote quality in organizations in the United States. Originally the award for performance excellence was targeted toward business; however, in 1995 a pilot project for healthcare and education was launched. In 1998, revised criteria for education and healthcare were developed and are available from the National Institute of Standards and Technology (NIST). Finally, in 1999, the award was made available to healthcare organizations.

Deming's philosophies and famous "14 Points for Management" are outlined in his books, *Out of the Crisis* and *The New Economics.* Many of Deming's philosophies are even older than his books and his 1950 presentation to the Japanese. Deming credits Walter Shewhart with many of the tools and techniques he introduced as integral to quality improvement. For example, the Plan, Do, Study, Act Cycle introduced later in this book that is frequently called the Deming Cycle was called the

Shewhart Cycle by Deming. Shewhart also developed the first control charts in the 1920s. At that time, he was a physicist with Bell Labs. He used control charts to analyze variation over time.

Although Deming and Shewhart made tremendous contributions to the field of quality, they certainly were not alone. In 1954, J. M. Juran was also invited to Japan where he presented a series of lectures on quality. Much of Juran's emphasis centered on management's responsibility to achieve quality. In later years, he founded The Juran Institute, and published the well-known book, *Juran's Quality Control Handbook,* along with several other popular books. Another innovator was Philip Crosby, who explored the area of the cost of quality. His book, *Quality is Free,* became an immediate success when it was published in 1979. The Japanese have also made great contributions to the field of quality. A Japanese man named Ishikawa is famous for inventing the Ishikawa Diagram (also known as the fishbone or cause-and-effect diagram). Ishikawa invented the diagram in 1943 to help organizations discover the root causes of problems. Taguchi is known for inventing the Taguchi Methods, which present ways to design experiments to improve quality. Both of these Japanese-originated methods are widely used in the United States today.

Quality Assurance vs. Performance Improvement

Traditionally, healthcare has emphasized Quality Assurance (QA). One of the main reasons for this was that in the past, JCAHO placed a great deal of importance on QA. Several years ago, JCAHO changed its standards to reflect an emphasis on PI rather than QA. Unfortunately, many healthcare organizations have not made the transition to PI. They are still expending a tremendous amount of energy meeting QA objectives, without getting the benefits that PI yields. The traditional QA is much different than PI. The QA focus is not on the "big picture" of continuously improving the way things are done, but rather on choosing specific things to monitor and regularly checking for compliance. There is a place for some of the initial QA efforts; however, the emphasis of organizations today should be on PI in order to reflect the current JCAHO standards. Look at the differences between the two and see where your organization falls.

The following chart gives some examples of the primary differences between QA and PI with further discussion afterward.

Quality Assurance	Performance Improvement
QA is defined as conformance to standards.	PI is defined as continuously improving organizational performance.
QA relies heavily on inspection—generally "after the fact" (i.e., record review).	Tools such as control charts are used to monitor ongoing processes and outcomes.
Individual items are separated from their process/system.	There is a system orientation.
Quality is a separate function in the organization.	Quality is integrated into all aspects of the organization.
Things are done departmentally or functionally.	Things are done in an interdisciplinary manner.

Quality Assurance	Performance Improvement
QA is defined as conformance to standards.	PI is defined as continuously improving organizational performance.

In the past, healthcare organizations involved in QA would generally set "thresholds" for things they wanted to measure. For example, a department might decide that during a certain period of time, it would expect 20 medication errors. Medication error data were then gathered and plotted on a chart next to the threshold value. If the department had fewer than 20 medication errors for each time period it was in great shape. If it had more, it knew that it had better take action before JCAHO came to visit. One of those actions may be to "raise the threshold" because the threshold was often just an arbitrary number anyway! Consequently, hospitals often set thresholds that they could easily meet and would get in trouble only if things got worse than expected. PI does not set arbitrary thresholds, but rather looks at past data trends and expectations of the customer—in this case the patient. For example, how many medication errors would the patient expect? Obviously zero! Therefore, the emphasis is placed on understanding the present system, and then taking steps to improve quality.

In the days of QA, one would rarely improve a process just to do it. Organizations waited to make changes until there were enough complaints to justify a change, or until something was clearly not working and/or costing too much money. The emphasis in PI is to look for ways to improve processes throughout the organization, and once a process is improved, to continue to look for ways to improve it.

Quality Assurance	Performance Improvement
QA relies heavily on inspection—generally "after the fact" (i.e., record review).	Tools such as control charts are used to monitor ongoing processes and outcomes.

Healthcare organizations involved in QA generally conducted extensive patient chart reviews—usually after the patient was discharged from the hospital. The records were reviewed to see if there were any *mistakes.* Although there is still a place for this type of a review in PI, part of the problem with this is that the patient is already gone and problems cannot be easily corrected. Performance improvement uses tools and techniques to monitor systems and processes as they occur. If there is a problem, it will be identified quickly and corrected without a long time delay. Therefore, the emphasis is on ongoing review, with retrospective review as a supplemental concern.

Quality Assurance	Performance Improvement
Individual items are separated from their process/system.	There is a system orientation.

As mentioned previously, the QA *threshold* method separated items from the system in which they worked, and measured these items independently. This disparate measurement process does not recognize that everything that occurs in a healthcare organization is part of a bigger process or system, and in order to affect the individual measurement, the system itself must be analyzed. JCAHO has identified the need for a "systems approach" in standards that expect that hospitals have a systematic approach to continuous improvement. For example, if the medication error rate increases, the entire system is examined for possible causes, rather than just dismissing it as *pharmacy's fault* or *nursing's fault.* The system approach even extends to the way changes are made. If one department decides to change a form there is an effort made to obtain feedback from all those affected by the change before the change is implemented.

One of the first things we did in QA was to find out who was to blame when a mistake was made. Often, if we couldn't find anyone to blame, there were no actions taken to correct the situation. PI follows an entirely different orientation. Deming noted that employees should be blamed for problems generally about 15 percent of the time. The remainder of the time, the problem is the fault of the system that allowed the mistake to occur in the first place. The idea behind PI is to change the system so quality is *built in* and it is difficult for individuals to make mistakes.

Quality Assurance	Performance Improvement
Quality is a separate function in the organization.	Quality is integrated into all aspects of the organization.

Often, what occurred in the QA approach was that hospitals would designate a Quality Department to handle quality issues. Quality then became the responsibility of this department, and everyone else just left it to the *quality people.* The idea of PI is that quality is the responsibility of everyone, and training is provided throughout the organization to help individuals learn the proper tools and techniques to improve quality. In PI, there may still be a quality department; however, this department provides training, expertise, and assistance to help others continuously improve their own processes.

Quality Assurance	Performance Improvement
Things are done departmentally or functionally.	Things are done in an interdisciplinary manner.

Whereas QA was often department or function oriented, PI emphasizes cross-function involvement. JCAHO has several standards that designate that organizational activities be interdisciplinary and carried out collaboratively. Organizations will demonstrate an interdisciplinary approach by having multiple departments represented on teams, providing meeting minutes that show input from various areas throughout the organization, and by showing documents such as flowcharts that span multiple functions/areas. JCAHO has especially emphasized an interdisciplinary approach when the organization is designing new processes or redesigning an existing process.

Quality: Been There . . . Done That . . .

Unfortunately, quality has become a bad word in some organizations. The quality assurance initiatives were many healthcare organizations' first foray into quality. These initiatives were often accompanied with little training and often failed. Once quality improvement came on the scene, some organizations rushed into QI initiatives with lots of enthusiasm. Bolstered by success stories in the media and books touting "free quality," quality became the next big thing to sweep the United States. Unfortunately, studies have shown that approximately two-thirds of all quality initiatives fail or are abandoned. With those odds, why should any organization implement quality improvement? The stunning results of the organizations that have successfully implemented quality improvement are enough to drive us forward. Healthcare organizations have the additional impetus of regulatory and accreditation requirements requiring some form of PI. As long as we have to do PI anyway, it makes sense to get as much out of it as possible.

Change is incredibly difficult. Any individual who tries once to change or improve and then gives up is considered a quitter. Sometimes it takes several tries to get it right. The same is true for organizations. If your healthcare organization has tried "quality" and it failed—learn from your mistakes and try again. When you succeed, it will be well worth your efforts.

Why Measurement Is Important

Earlier in the chapter it was mentioned that quality improvement efforts are data driven. What does that mean? In the past, organizations have often made decisions based on intuition or feelings. There is a place for intuition and feelings—but in quality, that place is as a complement to data and facts. For example, we may think that patients are unhappy with the way we provide a certain service. We may base this decision on our observations of the patients. We may then change the way we provide the service in order to make it more user–friendly. We may then observe later that patients appear to be happier. Although the intentions behind this are good, there are some problems with the implementation. For example, how do we know that the patients were truly unhappy with our service to begin with? How do we know that the changes we made actually improved the service to the patients? An example of intuition and data-driven quality improvement combined would be that intuition might prompt us to do a survey to determine patient satisfaction levels. This will give us baseline data. Now we know what level of satisfaction exists for our patients so that once we make changes, we can tell if the changes made any difference in the patients' satisfaction level. We will get input from the patients and employees alike to plan the change. Once the change is implemented, we will gather data to see if the change was positive. If it was, we will standardize the change and continue to improve the process over time. If the change was not positive, we will continue to examine what changes need to be made.

Integral to the preceeding process is measurement. *Measurement* is assessing the degree to which something is present. The *something* is whatever we are measuring. For example, if a healthcare organization is measuring patient satisfaction, it will measure the degree to which "satisfaction is present." This book explores various measurement techniques that are used in order to improve organizational performance.

Measurement Fundamentals

Attribute and Variable Data

What are *data*? Data are pieces of unprocessed information that are generally gathered or obtained in some way. There are two types of data. Data are either *attribute* or *variable*. Attribute data are things that are often considered *countable*; whereas variable data are things that are measured. The number of surgical complications is something we would count, rather than measure. The time a patient waits to see the physician is variable data because time is something we measure. Some examples of variable and attribute data are shown in the following chart.

Attribute Data	Variable Data
Number of surgical complications	Wait times in the clinic
Number of patients in the hospital	Dollar amount of accounts receivable
Number of delinquent patient charts	Actual surgical time less scheduled surgical time

This distinction is important when using control charts because the type of data being used (attribute or variable) will determine the type of control chart that is necessary. This concept—along with practice exercises—will be expanded on later in the book.

Data Gathering

The way data are gathered and the type of data that are gathered are very important in the measurement process. The Joint Commission has many standards that deal specifically with data gathering. For example, one of the PI standards refers to data being systematically collected. Systematic collection of data requires that data that are to be analyzed together be gathered in the same manner each time. Let's say that we want to see if the patient satisfaction levels are the same at each of our two clinics. If written surveys are given to the patients in Clinic 1 and verbal interviews are conducted in Clinic 2, there may be a difference in patient satisfaction levels. Unfortunately, because the data were not gathered systematically, it is difficult to determine if the difference is due to the way the data were gathered, or due to a true difference in satisfaction levels. Later in the book when checklists and operational definitions are discussed, this topic will be further explored.

Another aspect of interest to the Joint Commission involves sampling. When data are gathered there is a critical choice to make. One of the first things to determine is whether it is best to gather *population* or *sample data*. When we deal with a population it means that data are gathered from everyone or everything of interest. If sample data are obtained it means that data are gathered from a subset of the population. For example, if someone is doing a surgical case review, that person has the choice of looking at all of the surgical case records (population), or some of the surgical case records (sample).

Often, population data are difficult, if not impossible, to gather. Obviously, a patient satisfaction survey may be mailed to the population, but the respondents will most likely comprise a sample, as it is unlikely that everyone in the population will respond. Other times, population data are the only acceptable data to be gathered. For example, JCAHO requires that data regarding all confirmed transfusion reactions be gathered, as well as all significant adverse drug reactions. Obviously, sample data will not work—population data must be gathered in these circumstances.

As with most everything, there are advantages and disadvantages to each method.

> Population data are more accurate, but generally are more time-consuming and difficult to gather.
>
> Sample data are less accurate, but generally are less time-consuming and easier to gather.

Another element that enters into the sampling decision is how to choose the sample. There are many options to choose from; however, three of the most common are provided here.

Simple Random Sample

A simple random sample is generally considered one of the most credible of samples. The test for determining if a sample is truly a simple random sample is to ask if each item in the population had an equal probability of being included in the sample. In order to assure that this is the case, personal judgment cannot enter into the sampling decision. The method that removes the personal judgment often involves the use of a random number table or a computerized random number generator to identify the items to be chosen for the sample. Random number tables may be found in statistics books or may be generated from a calculator or computer program that has the appropriate capabilities. A random number table is simply a list of numbers that have been obtained in such a way that each number listed had an equal probability of being chosen. An example of the use of a random number table may involve the necessity of gathering a random sample of 100 of the healthcare organization's employees. In this case, we could take the first three numbers of each employee's social security number, refer to a random number table, and choose the first 100 employees who match numbers with the random number table. Sometimes the use of a preprinted random number table is not necessary. Many computer programs have the ability to choose a random sample by randomly selecting records that already exist in the computer.

Systematic Sample

A systematic sample is frequently used in healthcare and has a good deal of credibility. We say that in systematic sampling, every "*n*th" item is chosen to be in the sample. If we are reviewing patient records, we may choose every eleventh or twentieth record as listed alphabetically or in some other logical order. In order to increase the credibility of this method, an element of randomization may be added. This is done by choosing the starting point (the point at which the counting begins) randomly (by using a random number table).

Judgment Sample

A judgment sample is obtained by using our own discretion to choose items for the sample. This type of sample has very little credibility and is subject to bias. Although this is one of the most frequently used sampling methods, it is generally discouraged. It is often just as easy to choose a random or systematic sample as a judgment sample. Whenever possible, the systematic, random, or other credible methods should be used.

Summary

The quality journey is a rewarding one. It's not easy, and is often fraught with difficulties; however, the rewards are great for those organizations that embark on quality improvement. The remainder of this book will provide the tools and techniques to assist organizations in improving organizational performance.

EXERCISE

Step 1: Think about the way your organization addresses Performance Improvement. Review each category given here and perform one of the following options.

Option 1: In a group with others from your organization, discuss each category and determine where your organization falls in relationship to QA/PI. After discussing each category, agree on a score for each item.

Option 2: Individually think about each category in relationship to your organization. Determine a score that represents where your organization is now, and on a separate sheet of paper, write down specific examples that support your score.

Score Key:

1— Our activities are always QA

2— Our activities are primarily QA, with occasional PI initiatives

3— Our activities fall halfway between QA and PI

4— Our activities are primarily PI with occasional QA initiatives

5— Our activities are always PI

Quality Assurance	Performance Improvement
QA is defined as conformance to standards.	PI is defined as continuously improving organizational performance.

Our score in the area above is: 1 2 3 4 5

Quality Assurance	Performance Improvement
QA relies heavily on inspection—generally "after the fact" (i.e., record review).	Tools such as control charts are used to monitor ongoing processes and outcomes.

Our score in the area above is: 1 2 3 4 5

Quality Assurance	Performance Improvement
Individual items are separated from their process/system.	There is a system orientation.

Our score in the area above is: 1 2 3 4 5

Quality Assurance	Performance Improvement
Quality is a separate function in the organization.	Quality is integrated into all aspects of the organization.

Our score in the area above is: 1 2 3 4 5

Quality Assurance	Performance Improvement
Things are done departmentally or functionally.	Things are done in an interdisciplinary manner.

Our score in the area above is: 1 2 3 4 5

Step 2: Think about (or discuss) the areas that scored the lowest. What steps can be taken to move the organization toward PI?

References

Crosby, P. B. 1979. *Quality is Free.* New York: McGraw-Hill.

Deming, W. E. 1994. *The New Economics.* Cambridge, MA: Massachusetts Institute of Technology.

Deming, W. E. 1986. *Out of the Crisis.* Cambridge, MA: Massachusetts Institute of Technology.

Ishikawa, K. 1985. *What is Total Quality Control? The Japanese Way.* Englewood Cliffs, NJ: Prentice-Hall.

Juran, J. J. 1981. *Management of Quality,* 4th ed. Wilton, CT: Juran Institute.

Juran, J. J., and Gryna, F. M. 1988. *Juran's Quality Control Handbook,* 4th ed. New York: McGraw-Hill.

Taguchi, G. 1987. *Systems of Experimental Design.* Nagaya, Japan: UNIPUB.

CHAPTER 2

Getting Started in Quality in Healthcare

It is important that organizations identify a quality methodology. The methodology guides the individuals in the organization in continuous improvement. One of the most common methodologies adopted by organizations is known as the Shewhart Cycle; Deming Cycle; Plan, Do, Check, Act (PDCA) Cycle; or Plan, Do, Study, Act (PDSA) Cycle. Although it has many different names, the cycle is basically the same. Visually, the cycle looks like this:

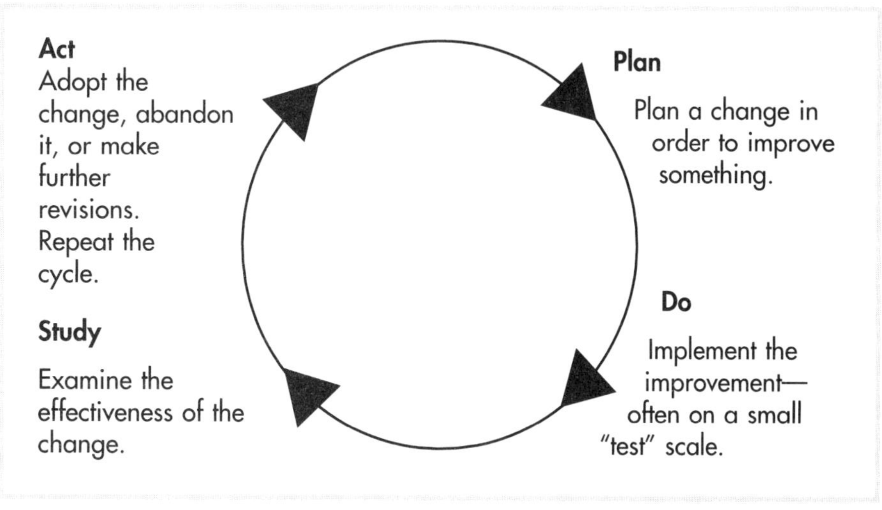

Act
Adopt the change, abandon it, or make further revisions. Repeat the cycle.
Plan
Plan a change in order to improve something.
Do
Implement the improvement—often on a small "test" scale.
Study
Examine the effectiveness of the change.

Source: Deming, 1995

This cycle has been adopted by many healthcare organizations as the *way they do performance improvement.* The circular element of the methodology shows the continuous improvement inherent in the process. One of the questions that JCAHO surveyors frequently ask employees during a survey is, What approach is used to improve existing processes? The PDSA Cycle is one such approach.

Leadership and Quality

The discussion of leadership and quality could be a book in and of itself. Therefore, the topic is briefly mentioned here with specific references to JCAHO's requirements; however, it is recommended that any leader on the road to quality should study the topic in much more detail than is provided here.

Although one of the primary drivers for implementing QI is generally the requirements by regulatory and insurance agencies, this doesn't stop many successful leaders from embracing quality and making it their own. Numerous studies, regarding the reasons why quality implementation has failed in organizations, have shown that the lack of committed, visible leadership ranks as one of the most common reasons for failure.

For example, if quality training occurs and the top management does not attend, it sends a clear signal that leadership has relegated quality to the "lower ranks." In these circumstances, often the employees view the new training as "flavor of the month" and do the bare minimum while waiting for the quality initiative to die out as other programs have done in the past. It is up to management to say and show that this is different. Quality is not a passing fad—it is the way we do things.

One mistake that is often made by management is to add layers of new, quality-related systems and processes on top of existing systems. This creates unnecessary or duplicative processes and results in confusion and a waste of precious resources. Obviously, there is resistance from employees when this is done because it stretches people even further. The response is, "When am I supposed to find the time for these new things you want me to do?" Instead, we need to examine the things that exist from the old QA structure that can be removed, and present QI/PI as a way to find even more efficiencies while increasing quality.

Another mistake that is made is for management to ignore the training needs of employees. Although employees in some departments have been trained in the use of statistical methods because of the nature of their educational degrees, the approaches to measurement in most healthcare areas have been less than scientific. The very essence of QI is founded on a statistical, data-driven approach. This can be scary for people not accustomed to using these methods. Research has shown that training is critical for successful QI implementation.

It is not enough, however, to train all employees and think that QI will then naturally follow. Beginning with, and immediately following the training, employees should be given structured opportunities to use the QI tools in real situations. For example, during a training session regarding the use of an Ishikawa diagram, employees should come prepared to perform the Ishikawa steps with a real problem in the organization. Following the training, the employees should be placed in a group to tackle another problem using the Ishikawa diagram. It is also important that a resource person is identified so that if groups have questions regarding the use of the tools they can get assistance.

In 1999, JCAHO made a change to its standards that had a dramatic effect upon leadership. In the past when there were problems with quality, leadership was only mildly affected in the scoring of the standards. In 1999, JCAHO put the scoring emphasis for quality in the leadership section of the standards. Therefore, an organization that is not successfully implementing QI will not do well in its leadership scores. Changing the culture of an organization from a compliance mentality to a QI mentality is not easy and takes an enormous amount of time and effort. However, the only way these changes will be effective is if leadership is firmly behind the initiatives.

The Performance Improvement (PI) Plan

Many healthcare organizations already have a quality plan or quality manual, as it is one of the requirements of JCAHO. JCAHO refers to this plan as the *Performance Improvement Plan*—or PI Plan. Often the plan is developed and placed on the shelf until it is dusted off for a visit by a regulatory agency. Even though a quality plan/manual may already exist, the development of a new one is actually a good place to start when an organization is creating an organizational culture that embraces continuous performance improvement. As long as the plan has to exist anyway—it makes sense to make it a working, living document.

What is the purpose of having a plan in the first place? Plans are generally used to state and clarify policies and procedures in a formalized, standardized manner. Therefore, a PI Plan describes the healthcare organization's procedures regarding quality and the quality methodology the organization has adopted to improve its organizational performance. Think of a group of people pushing a large boulder in different directions. This often happens in organizations when everyone is acting independently. It is frequently necessary to develop a unifying vision in order to obtain constancy of purpose. A PI Plan will help in this area. The PI Plan should also be closely aligned and integrated with the strategic plan, regulatory standards, and contractual quality obligations.

The steps in developing a PI Plan follow.

Form an interdisciplinary team.

↓

Present timetable for management approval.

↓

Review strategic plan, regulatory standards, and contractual obligations.

↓

Benchmark other quality manuals and plans.

↓

Determine and outline sections of the plan.

↓

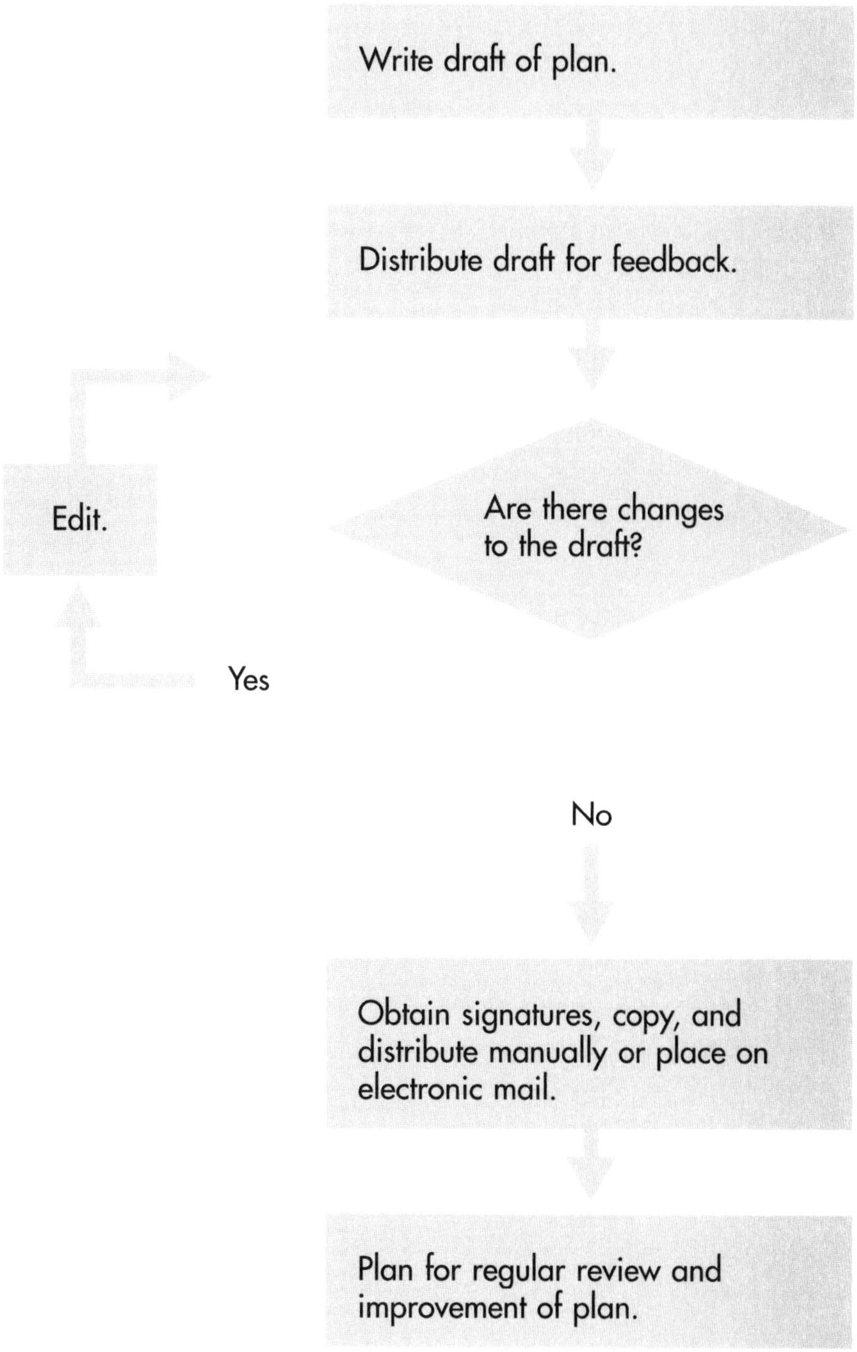

Write draft of plan.

Distribute draft for feedback.

Are there changes to the draft?

Yes

Edit.

No

Obtain signatures, copy, and distribute manually or place on electronic mail.

Plan for regular review and improvement of plan.

Form an interdisciplinary team.

↓

JCAHO places a strong emphasis on interdisciplinary approaches—and for good reason. It is important to gain input from diverse representatives of the organization. If the team that develops the PI Plan is composed of people solely from administration, it decreases the *buy-in* factor from the other departments. Try to get a cross section of employees on the plan development team. It also helps to include *informal leaders* in the organization—those who have the respect of their peers. Don't forget that you also need some people on the team who have good writing skills!

Present timetable for management approval.

↓

Unless the leadership of the writing team is very good, it is easy for a team to languish. A schedule will help keep the team on track and will also keep management informed of the status of the plan along the way. A sample schedule follows. (Figure 2.1) Notice that this schedule is slightly more detailed than the flowchart. The flowchart is a *macro* chart that shows the major steps; whereas, the schedule shows a more detailed view of the process.

Review strategic plan, regulatory standards, and contractual obligations.

↓

The PI Plan should naturally flow from the strategic plan. One of the first steps is to review the strategic plan and determine strategic quality objectives. These should be considered and referred to throughout the development of the PI Plan. Regulatory standards and contractual obligations should also be reviewed for their requirements regarding quality. These will often determine items to be included in the plan, such as measurable quality objectives.

	JAN				FEB				MAR				APR				MAY				...	
WEEK:	**1**	**2**	**3**	**4**	**1**	**2**	**3**	**4**	**1**	**2**	**3**	**4**	**1**	**2**	**3**	**4**	**1**	**2**	**3**	**4**		
Review strategic plan, regulatory standards and contractual obligations																						
Gather benchmark data																						
Review benchmark data																						
Determine sections, outline plan																						
Obtain approval for sections																						
Write draft of plan																						
Proof draft																						
Obtain feedback of draft																						
Revise draft																						
Obtain feedback of final proof																						
Obtain signatures																						
Print/copy plan																						
Distribute plan																						

Figure 2.1 A PI Plan.

Benchmark other quality manuals and plans.

Benchmarking is a term that refers to the process of looking for organizations that "do what you do," only better—and then imitating them. In this case, rather than creating a PI Plan from ground zero, review the PI Plans of other organizations to save time, effort, and money. After obtaining copies of other PI Plans, choose the *best of the best* to include in your plan—then rewrite those sections in your own words. JCAHO provides copies of two such plans in their IOP courses conducted regularly around the country. Your local or state hospital/healthcare association may also have access to plans for you to review. But you don't have to limit yourself to hospital plans—many businesses also have quality manuals that are very similar to PI Plans. You can look for manuals/plans both inside healthcare and outside of healthcare. One cautionary note—in order to make the plan truly yours, do not copy some other organization's PI Plan *verbatim* with the only change being the name of the healthcare organization. This defeats the intent and the spirit of the PI Plan (it is also called plagiarism!).

Determine and outline sections of the plan.

A sample outline of possible sections is as follows:

I. Introduction
   a. Purpose
   b. PI objectives
II. Guiding statements
   a. Mission
   b. Goals
   c. Core values
   d. Measurable objectives that are aligned with strategic plan, regulatory agencies, and/or contractual obligations
III. Systematic approach to performance improvement

a. Dimensions of performance (JCAHO)
b. PI methodology
c. New process design/process redesign

IV. Deployment of PI Plan
a. Teams
b. Training
c. Resources
d. Quality responsibilities of leadership and staff
e. Establishment of PI priorities

V. Evaluation
a. Measuring results
b. Root cause analysis
c. Assessing the results
d. Communication of quality results
e. Annual evaluation and improvement of the PI Plan

VI. Other
a. Confidentiality
b. Conflict of interest
c. Immunity from liability
d. Retention of records
e. Role in risk management

VII. Signatures

VIII. Forms/Attachments
a. Performance improvement team proposal form
b. Criteria for performance improvement priority form
c. Organization-wide measurement activities
d. PI flowchart

It is recommended that once you determine the sections of your plan you obtain management feedback and approval on the sections.

Write draft of plan.

One of the first things you want to do is to agree on a word processing software package that the plan will be written in. Next, you can assign sections to various people for writing. Remember that unless you obtain permission from the owners of the plans you benchmarked, you can't take what they wrote and copy it verbatim into your plan. You can, however, take their concepts and rewrite them accordingly. Your team may want to assign one proofreader who will read everything as it is written and make changes. One proofreader will give the document continuity. Once the section is written, the disk and paper copy will go to the proofreader. Generally, it helps if the proofreader has permission from the team to make the changes directly on the disks as he or she receives the sections. The proofreader is also the one who will assemble all the sections into the draft as they are received.

The team will also need to make several decisions at this point. The questions that follow should be answered by the team prior to the writing.

1. What will our section numbering system be?
2. How will we number tables/figures/charts?
3. What will our margins/font size/font be?
4. What will our writing style be?
5. How many spaces will our indentations be?
6. How will our headings be identified (i.e., bold, underlined, etc.)
7. Will we have any headers/footers? If so, what? Where?

Distribute draft for feedback.

Again, remember to distribute the plan draft to a cross section of people for feedback. Give them a time frame in which to read the plan, and follow up with reminders. In order to obtain feedback, ask them to write their suggestions on the plan. You may want to double-space this draft to make room for suggestions. You will get the best feedback by bringing the readers together in a meeting at which time they bring their written changes, and you can ask for additional feedback. This serves two purposes—it helps the readers to complete the reading on time and it also gathers ideas the readers may not want to take the time to write down, but will give freely in a discussion atmosphere.

Are there changes to the draft?

If there are changes to the draft—and there should be unless you are perfection personified—you will discuss the changes as a team. Try not to be defensive at this point, and take all suggestions with an open mind. Make all changes you agree on and distribute the plan again to either the same people or different people. If you distribute the plan to the same people, include a cover sheet that discusses any changes you did not make and the reasons you did not make them. You may have to repeat these review steps several times until you have obtained consensus.

Obtain signatures, copy, and distribute manually or place on electronic mail.

Once the plan is complete, you will obtain the appropriate signatures (JCAHO recommends the Administrator/CEO, President of the Medical Staff, and Chair of the Board of Directors). When you distribute the plan, keep a distribution list, because as you make changes, you will need to forward copies of the revisions to all plan holders so they may update their copies. Of course, if you can place the plan on electronic mail, you have eliminated the need for all of the paper updates and paper copies because as you make changes, you will automatically update the plan on the system.

Plan for regular review and improvement of plan.

Continuous improvement also applies to the plan itself. As your organization changes, the plan should change. Build in a regular review process and continue to improve the plan over time.

Now that we've covered many of the first steps in the quality journey, the following chapters will provide the how-to steps in beginning to use control charts.

EXERCISE

If available, review your organization's PI Plan. If the plan is not available, reflect upon your knowledge of your organization's PI Plan. If no PI Plan exists, think about what internal structures guide the organization when answering the following questions.

1. What is our quality methodology—how do we *do performance improvement*?
2. If everyone in the organization were asked to describe the organization's quality methodology, what would they say?
3. Is our PI Plan in alignment with our mission, vision, and values? If so, what specific things demonstrate that? If not, what is out of alignment? If no PI Plan exists, how do we communicate our mission, vision, and values to employees?
4. Does our PI Plan provide information regarding how we design new processes and redesign existing processes? If so, do we follow these guidelines across the organization? What are some examples of this? If not (or if no PI Plan exists), how do we design and redesign processes?
5. How are measurement and improvement priorities determined at our organization? Does the PI Plan give us guidance in this area? If so, do we use the guidance it provides?
6. How do we handle problem solving in our organization? Does the PI Plan guide us in a root cause analysis? If so, do we utilize the guidelines?
7. After answering the previous questions, do we believe the PI Plan (as it presently exists) is a useful tool in our organization? If not, what can we do to make it useful? If a PI Plan does not exist, how could it help us in the future?

Reference

Deming, W. E. 1986. *Out of the Crisis.* Cambridge, MA: Massachusetts Institute of Technology.

CHAPTER 3

Introduction to Control Charts

What Is a Control Chart?

A *control chart* is a graph that provides a pictorial representation of whatever it is you're measuring over a period of time and allows you to identify when special causes of variation are active in your process. If you have not worked with control charts before, you may not be familiar with *special causes of variation.* During the last few years, the JCAHO has added a standard regarding the identification of special causes of variation. One of the best ways to meet this standard is to use control charts. The discussion on variation that follows will help you to understand variation and its relationship to control charts.

Understanding Variation: The Key to Controlling Your Process

Variation is at the very heart of control charts. What do we mean by *variation*? An ancient philosopher once offered a reward for anyone who could make two loaves of bread that would turn out exactly the same. Obviously, it's impossible—and he knew it. He offered the reward to make a point about variability. The point is that variability is all around us. Think about the bread for a minute. You may use the exact same ingredients in both loaves, use the same oven, knead the dough the same amount of time—but you will get two different loaves of bread. Obviously, the system or the process used to make the two loaves of bread was exactly the same for both—but the process resulted in two different loaves of bread. Of course, that doesn't surprise us. We expect to have variability that will be reflected in slightly different loaves of bread. That variation is what a control chart is designed to capture. Conversely, what if you changed the oven temperature or kneaded one loaf longer than the other? Now, you would expect the loaves to be different because something in the system (or the process) has changed.

Think about the two differences you will find based on the two scenarios described. One difference is due to the changes made in the system. In other words, you treated the loaves differently because you kneaded one more than the other, or baked one at a higher temperature than the other. Deming called that *special cause variation.* The other difference is due to natural variability that we expect to occur in the system even though nothing has changed. Deming called that *common cause variation.* The exciting thing about control charts is they detect special cause variation, so you know if the changes you see day-to-day are due to common cause variation or due to a special cause upon the system.

Let's look at an example before we move on to expand this point even further. Figure 3.1 shows average monthly wait times for patients in the outpatient center. These times reflect the average amount of time that patients wait before seeing a physician. You'll note that the patient wait times began to increase in June. You may begin to worry, because in June you also hired a new director for the outpatient center. You wonder if the increase in wait times is due to the director. Now, think about what could happen in this situation.

Mistake 1: You think that it is special cause when it's really common cause.

If this happens, you think that the increase in wait time is due to the new director's actions—but in fact, you're mistaken. The increase in wait times is really just part of the natural (or common cause) variation in the system. Therefore, the director is getting blamed for something that he or she has not caused.

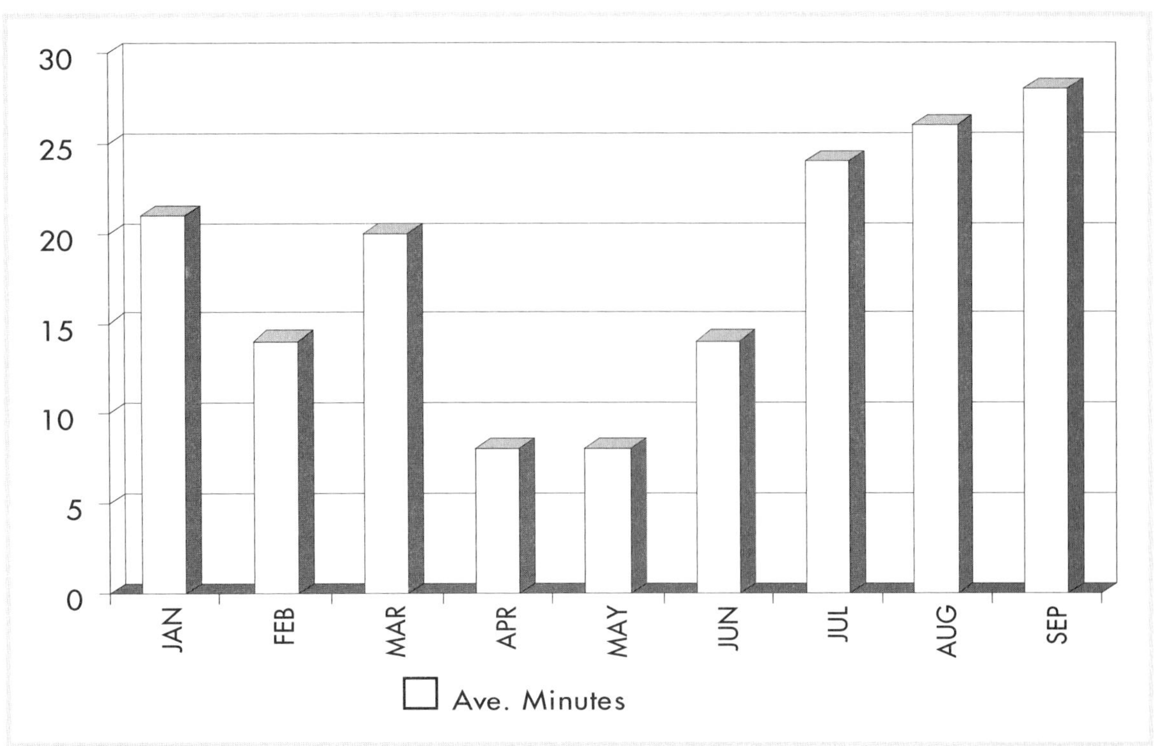

Figure 3.1. Average outpatient center patient wait times.

Mistake 2: You think that it is a common cause when it's really special cause.

If this happens, you think that the increase in wait time is just common cause variability in the system, when it's really due to the new director's actions. Therefore, the director should be held responsible for the changes he or she has made.

As you can see, the actions that one would take for common cause and special cause variation are different. When we have common cause variation, it is the variation that we expect to have—it is the variation that happens when we bake two loaves of bread using the same method each time. What are the actions we take in that situation? We might experiment with various bread pans or kneading methods—but we wouldn't get upset because the two loaves are different and start blaming the baker. We can either accept common cause variation, or we can make changes in the system to reduce the overall variation. In the outpatient center wait time example, if the variation was common cause, we know that even if wait times increase for a while, they will also decrease, because that's the variability that naturally happens in a system. If, however, the wait time is unacceptable, we can make changes to the system in order to reduce the common cause variation.

On the other hand, special cause (the oven is too hot, the bread was not kneaded long enough) warrants an investigation. Ultimately, we may determine that no long-term action is necessary because it probably won't happen again; however, it is still important to find out what happened that resulted in the special cause. In the bread example, perhaps a new employee turned the oven too high. If we hire new employees only once a year, there probably isn't a need to do sweeping orientation changes and initiate new workplace rules regarding the oven. However, if we hire new bakers once every few weeks, we may want to examine our training procedures to make sure the bakers learn the proper oven temperature. If it's a high-risk situation or extremely costly, we may want to take preventative action even though the special cause may not occur very often. A summary of these concepts is presented in Figure 3.2.

What It Is \ What You Think	**Common Cause**	**Special Cause**
Common Cause	You accurately determined that the variability existed in the system. You either leave it alone, or change the system to reduce the variability.	You mistakenly determined that the variability was due to a special cause. Your reaction/ change may have resulted in over-correction of the system.
Special Cause	You mistakenly determined that the variability existed in the system. You ignored it, and perhaps missed an opportunity for improvement.	You accurately determined that the variability was due to something outside the system or a change in the system. You identify the source and react if necessary.

Figure 3.2. Common and special cause variation.

So far, only negative examples have been presented (the wait time is too long, the oven is too hot, and so forth). However, what if we see improvements in the measurement? It is also important to determine if the improved measurements reflect common or special cause. If the wait times decreased, it would be important to determine if the changes were due to the new director, or if it is common cause variation, which will probably fluctuate and increase again in the near future.

Process Stability

JCAHO has several standards that relate to process stability. Organizations should be able to determine if their key processes are stable. This is a direct reference to common and special cause variation. When a process is *stable*, it is exhibiting common cause variation with no special cause variation. When a process is *unstable*, it has evidence of special cause variation. The best way to determine process stability is to use a control chart.

Control Chart Description

There are three very important lines on a control chart. Figure 3.3 shows that all control charts have an upper control limit (UCL), a center line (CL), and a lower control limit (LCL). The easiest way to explain a control chart is to give an example of its use. Let's say that our hospital outpatient center director wants to measure the average time that patients spend waiting to see a physician in the outpatient center. The center line of the control chart is the average time that patients wait to see the physician. The upper control limit and the lower control limit show the expected range of common cause variation within the process. The UCL is the upper limit assuming no special cause (for example, natural disaster emergency) occurs, and the LCL is the lower limit.

In this example, we will be plotting the sample means of actual wait times. Therefore, at our hospital, the average time that patients wait in the outpatient center is 18 minutes (CL), as reflected in Figure 3.4. The longest expected average time patients wait is 33 minutes (UCL), while the shortest time is 3 minutes (LCL). Once the control chart has been

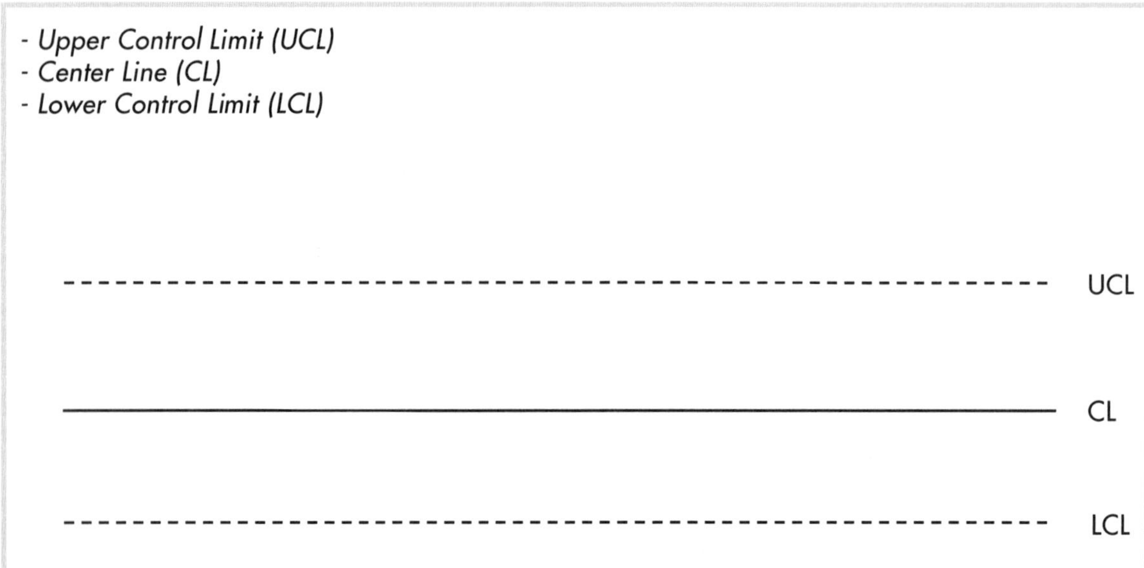

Figure 3.3. Elements of all control charts.

constructed as this one has, we can begin to gather data over a period of time in order to monitor the outpatient wait times. We used past data to develop the control chart shown in Figure 3.4. Figure 3.4 shows how we now view our patient wait time over a period of months. As you can see, control charts display data over time. In this case, we chose to display by month, but could have chosen to display the data by day, week, or any other time increment.

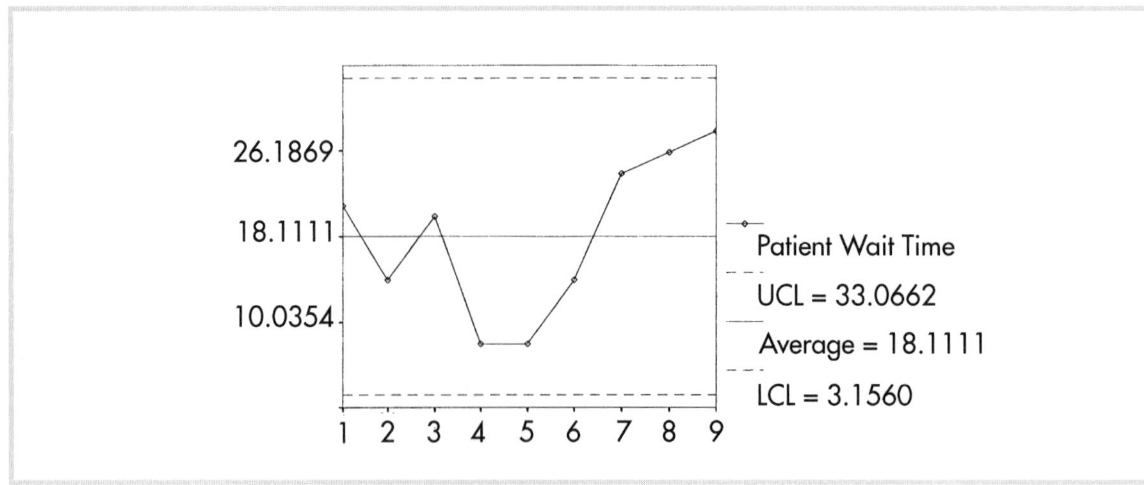

Figure 3.4. Control chart for patient wait times.

Control Chart History

One of the good things about control charts is that they have been used for a number of years and have been shown to be very effective. Control charts were developed by Walter Shewhart of Bell Laboratories in the early 1920s and were used originally at the Western Electric plant near Chicago. Edwards Deming popularized the use of control charts on a global level. Originally, control charts were used extensively in manufacturing applications; however, in the last 15 years, they have become widely used in service industries as well.

Control Chart Use in Healthcare

Control charts have direct applicability in healthcare. In fact, many of the Performance Improvement Standards from JCAHO can be met by using control charts. As mentioned earlier, there is a JCAHO standard that asks about common and special cause variation. In general, control charts have the following uses regarding data:

- Understanding
- Monitoring
- Improving
- Verifying

Understanding

Control charts are very useful to help understand a process and its capabilities. When developing the control chart, information is obtained about the average, the upper control limit, and the lower control limit of whatever is being measured. This provides an understanding of the performance and restraints of the system. For example, knowing that the average wait time in our outpatient center is 18 minutes, we would not readily sign a service provider agreement that promises an average wait time of 10 minutes unless we changed the system. The control chart shows that the system will simply not perform well enough to meet the 10-minute average unless changes are made in our procedures.

Monitoring

Control charts allow us to monitor things over time. Healthcare organizations may choose to use control charts to display data that they are required to gather for regulatory compliance, insurance companies, or for their own information. Organizations can also use control charts, particularly in high-risk areas, to provide ongoing, current information on the performance of the system, instead of discovering problems well after the fact. Control charts are useful to study the impact of various factors (that is, special causes) upon the measurements. For example, slightly different measurements may occur when the weather is particularly hot or cold—or perhaps even during a full moon.

Improving

Control charts can be used to improve the processes or systems in organizations. As the process is monitored, problems may be identified and improvement priorities may surface.

Verifying

Control charts are very helpful to verify if changes made to the system reflect in improved system performance. For example, a new form may be used to decrease the patient wait times. A control chart will show visually if the form is effective or not.

Interpreting Control Charts

With that in mind, there are several guidelines that help to interpret control charts. The guidelines provided here are considered general and will assist in most situations. There are many more guidelines than are presented in this book. The five that follow are generally the most commonly used. Once you are comfortable with control charts, you can begin to move into more sophisticated evaluation. More detailed guidelines are available from Statistical Process Control (SPC) books. Two such books are by Grant and Leavenworth, and Mitra. Complete references for these two books are provided at the end of this chapter. If you decide to move into more extensive evaluation in the future, you may also find that there is some disagreement in the literature about the evaluation rules. For example, some publications define a *trend* as seven consecutive increasing or decreasing points. Others have stated that a trend must contain eight, or even nine, consecutive points. This book presents the most widely held views; however, don't be surprised if you come across other viewpoints when you review other publications.

Since the control limits are based on the common cause variation of the process, a random display of points within the control limits should be evident. If this is true, we say that the process is *in statistical control*, which means that only common cause variation is active in the process. *This is what JCAHO refers to as a stable process.* If special cause variation becomes active, we will see a change in the random pattern or we will notice nonrandom patterns. When any of the following patterns are evident on our control chart, the process is *out-of-control. This is what JCAHO refers to as an unstable process.* If a process is deemed out-of-control it is not necessarily a negative situation. For example, the actions we take to decrease the patient wait times may result in a control chart that would be labeled out-of-control. In this case, it simply means that the changes that were made have made a difference, and it is likely that the control chart limits need to be recalculated. Each guideline is illustrated with an example from the outpatient center wait time situation.

1. Points Outside of the Control Limits (Figure 3.5)

   It is highly unlikely that a measurement will fall outside of the UCL or the LCL by chance if the process is in statistical control. When this occurs, it means that a special cause has influenced the system. For example, the computers in the outpatient center may be inoperable, causing a long delay at the registration desk.

2. A Run (Figure 3.6)

   A *run* occurs when seven or more consecutive points fall on either side of the center line. If the points fall above the center line in the wait time example, it is possible that the director has initiated changes that have "bumped up" the whole process in terms of time. Perhaps the average wait time has increased from 18 minutes to 20 minutes. Conversely, if the points fall below the center line, it is possible that the entire system has experienced a decrease in the average

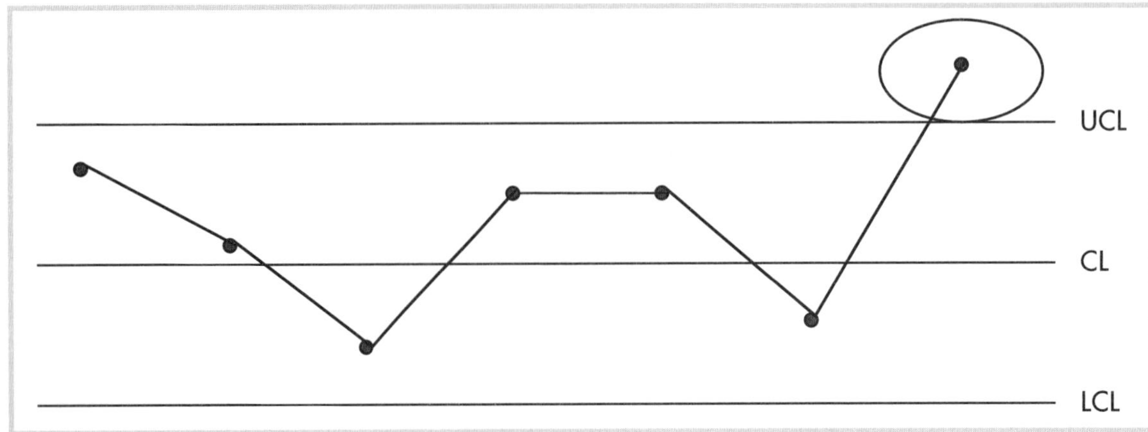

Figure 3.5. A point outside of control limits.

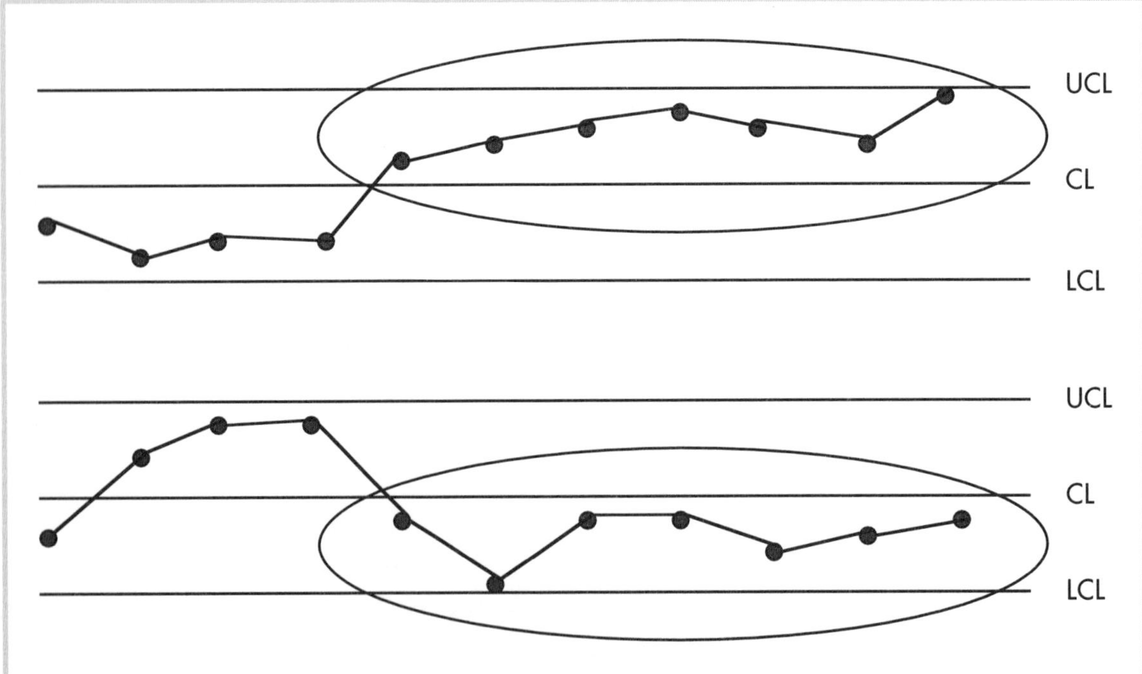

Figure 3.6. A run.

due to actions taken within the system. If the change is an improvement, we would want to make sure it is integrated into the standard operating instructions. If it was not an improvement, it would be important to identify the reason behind the special cause and eliminate it if possible. Whenever the common cause variation changes, we want to gather data to recalculate the control chart's CL, UCL, and LCL.

3. A Trend (Figure 3.7)

    When seven consecutive points move steadily upward or downward, it is forming a *trend.* In the example cited, if the trend was upward, it would indicate that the wait times were increasing. This is important to know because when most people look at a graph, they don't really know when to call the situation a trend, or when it is just an artifact of common cause variation. When there are seven consecutive points in the wait time example that are either increasing or decreasing, it may be possible that the director has indeed done something to influence the system (either positively or negatively, depending upon the direction of the trend). Keep in mind that in our first example, the data were displayed by month. It is likely that we may not want to wait seven months to see if there is a trend. It is possible to display the data by day or even week. Therefore, it is possible to determine if there is a trend much sooner than seven months.

4. Hugging the Center Line (Figure 3.8)

    If a control chart shows four out of five consecutive points that are near or at the center line, it is generally an indication of one of two things. One possibility is that the data are being manipulated

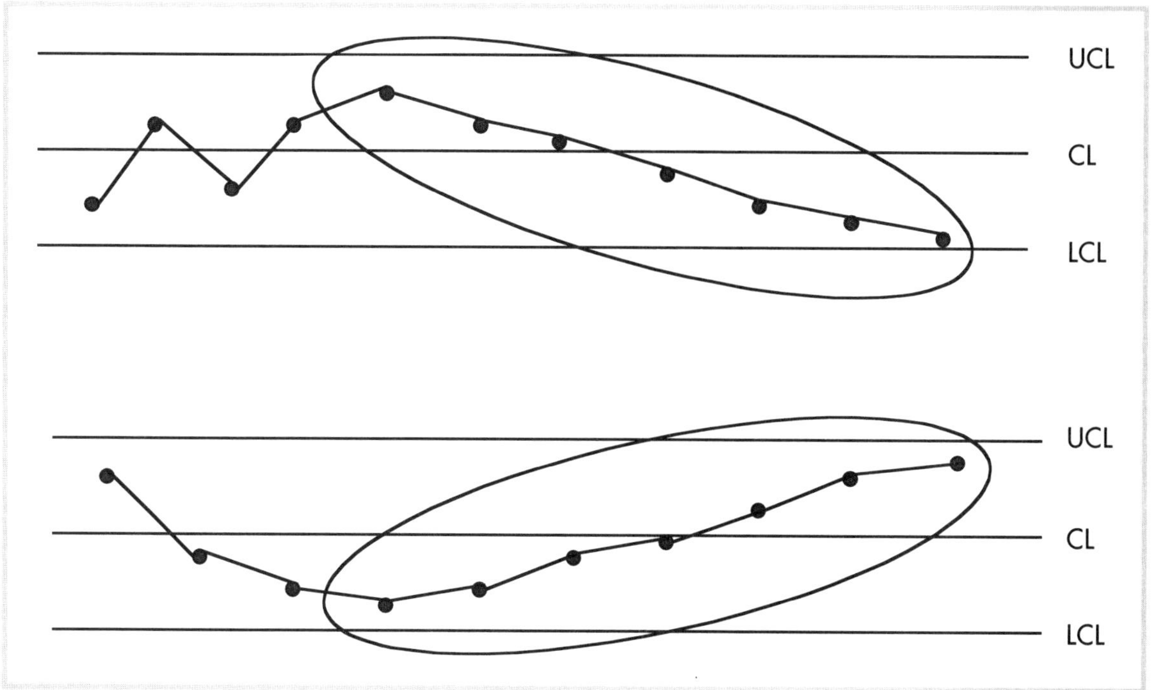

Figure 3.7. A trend.

or reported incorrectly, because the range of variability expected to occur is not occurring. On the positive side, the other possibility is that the variability within the system has been reduced, even though the mean has stayed the same.

Is it a good thing or a bad thing to reduce variability? Let me give an example to help you decide. I once took a month-long train trip. During this trip there were extensive employee labor problems and the trains were extremely unpredictable. The train could leave exactly on time, or could be hours late in leaving and/or arriving. Several of my connections were up to eight hours behind schedule. Obviously, if a control chart were used to measure the time the train departure deviated from the scheduled time, that control chart would show a lot of variability. In fact, the difference between the upper and lower control limit might be as great as 10 hours! Shortly after that train trip, I went to Japan and traveled on the bullet train. In comparison, the bullet train left and arrived on time almost to the minute. The control chart for the bullet train would show very little variability, with the distance between the upper and lower control limits perhaps as small as five minutes. It is evident in this situation the train with the least variability is the most desirable one. This holds true for most situations—one would be hard-pressed to find a process in which the process improves as the variability increases.

Now, let's say that while you were using a control chart for the train system with lots of variability, the labor problems were settled and the trains became more predictable. In other words, the change in the system resulted in reduced variability as evidenced by a control chart that *hugs the center line.* When this occurs, it is time to cel-

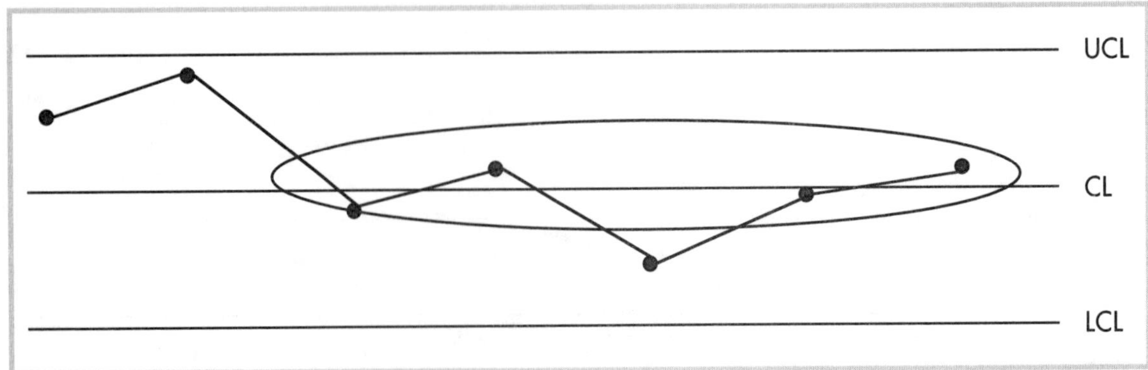

Figure 3.8. Hugging the center line.

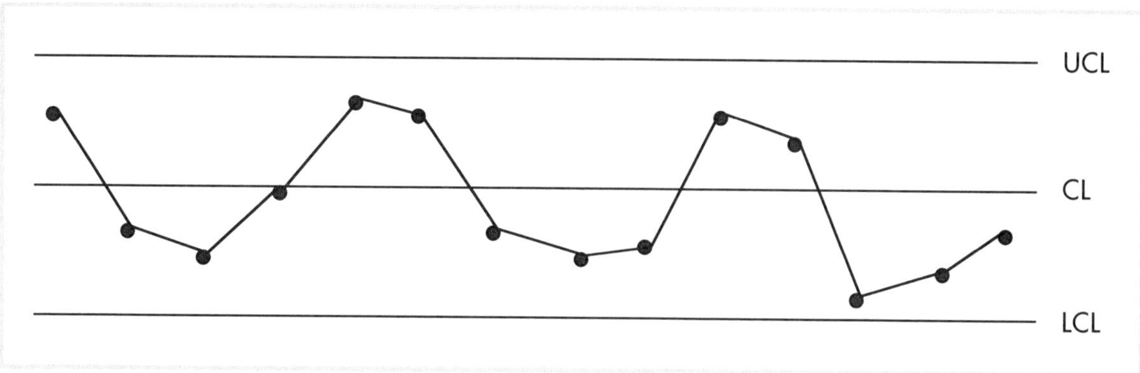

Figure 3.9. A cyclical pattern.

ebrate, and then recalculate the control chart limits to reflect the new limits.

5. A Cyclical Pattern (Figure 3.9)

   A repeating up-and-down pattern indicates that there is something systematic that is affecting the process. In the wait time example, it may be that every Monday and Friday the wait times increase because employees like to take those days off, resulting in short-staffing. Every Tuesday, Wednesday, and Thursday, the wait times decrease because the center has optimal staffing. In this situation, this pattern would not be evident on a monthly control chart, but would be evident if the control chart was updated daily. When patterns such as this exist, the random variation that is expected to occur is not happening—in other words, the common cause variation is not evident; instead a systematic pattern of variation shows that something is affecting the process.

These guidelines on interpreting control charts will be useful when you start developing your own control charts. Now that you know some of the guidelines, let's look again at the outpatient center's control chart in Figure 3.10.

In light of the guidelines discussed, and comparing the data with the control limits, we can see that there is no indication that the data from June onward is anything other than common cause variation. In an actual situation, it would also be important to review an additional control chart that shows the range or standard deviation before making a final decision. That concept is covered in the following chapter. At least initially, the data do not support the conjecture that the new director's policies have increased the patient wait times. On the other hand, it also does not show any improvement either.

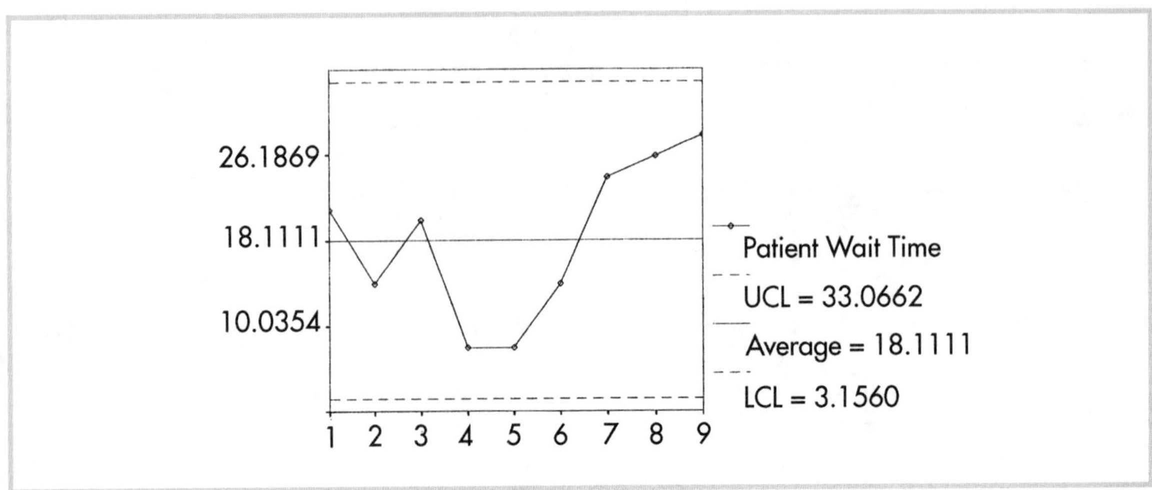

Figure 3.10. Control chart for patient wait times.

The following exercises will give you practice in interpreting control charts.

EXERCISES—INTERPRETING CONTROL CHARTS

INSTRUCTIONS

Look at each of the following control charts and determine if the variability is common cause or if there could be special cause variability present as reflected in an out-of-control chart. If the control chart is out-of-control, circle the applicable area and think of a situation this control chart could be measuring. Place hypothetical numbers for the CL, UCL, and LCL, and determine a possible cause and action for the situation the control chart is measuring.

1. Figure 3.11

   a. This control chart is ❑ in control *or stable* (go to next question)

      ❑ out-of-control *or unstable* (continue with this question)

   b. Specifically, the problem with this chart is: ________________

   c. This control chart could be measuring ________________

      ____

      ____

   d. The following could have caused this to occur ______________

      ____

      ____

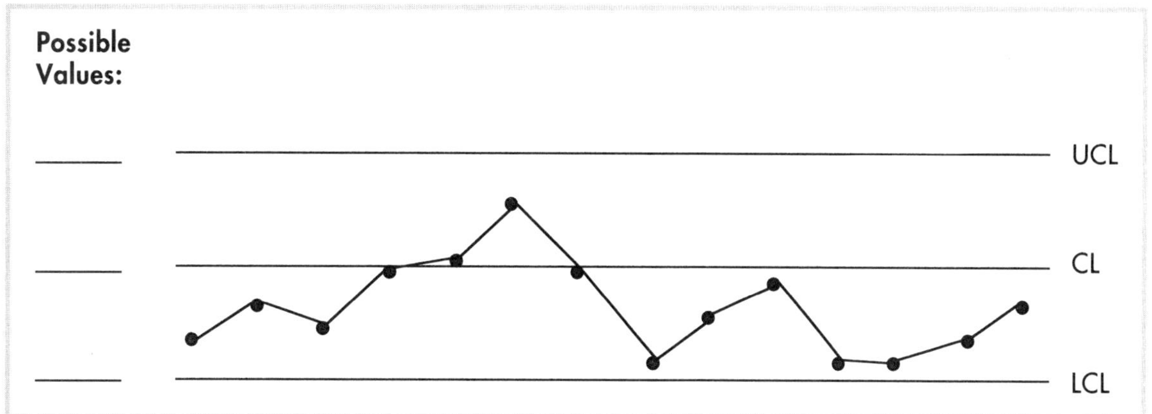

Figure 3.11.

e. We would recommend taking the following actions (no action is also an appropriate option if the situation is unlikely to repeat itself): ______________________________

____

____

2. Figure 3.12

a. This control chart is ❑ in control *or stable* (go to next question)

❑ out-of-control *or unstable* (continue with this question)

b. Specifically, the problem with this chart is: ______________

c. This control chart could be measuring ______________

____

____

d. The following could have caused this to occur ______________

____

____

e. We would recommend taking the following actions (no action is also an appropriate option if the situation is unlikely to repeat itself): ______________________________

____

____

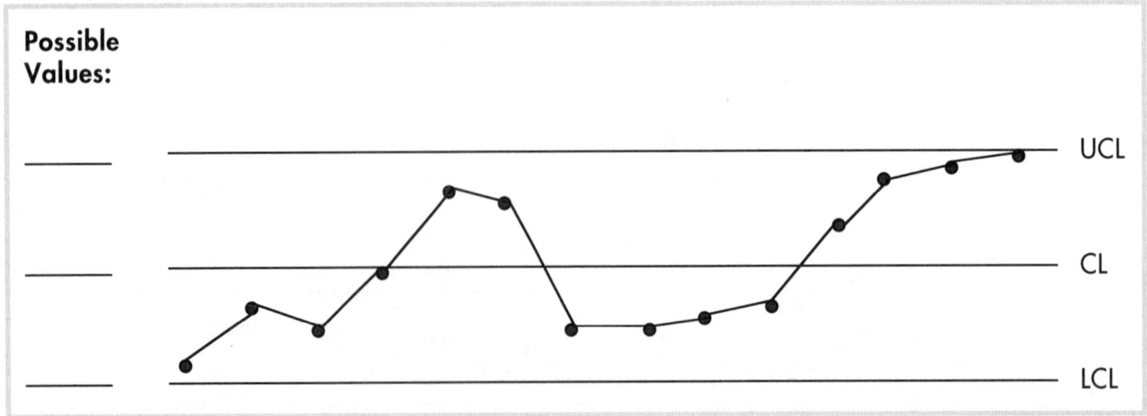

Figure 3.12.

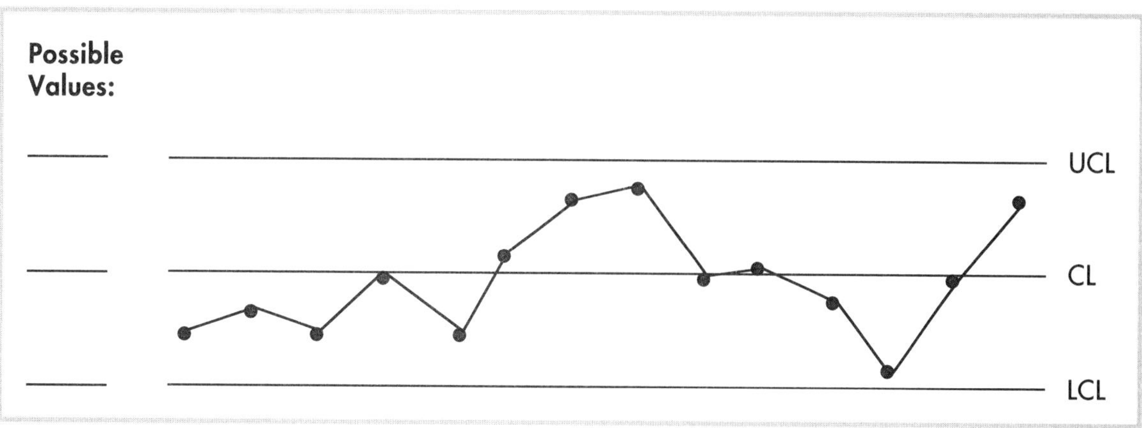

Figure 3.13.

3. Figure 3.13

   a. This control chart is ❑ in control *or stable* (go to next question)

      ❑ out-of-control *or unstable* (continue with this question)

   b. Specifically, the problem with this chart is: ______________

   c. This control chart could be measuring ______________

      ____

      ____

   d. The following could have caused this to occur ______________

      ____

      ____

   e. We would recommend taking the following actions (no action is also an appropriate option if the situation is unlikely to repeat itself): ______________

      ____

      ____

4. Figure 3.14

   a. This control chart is ❑ in control *or stable* (go to next question)

      ❑ out-of-control *or unstable* (continue with this question)

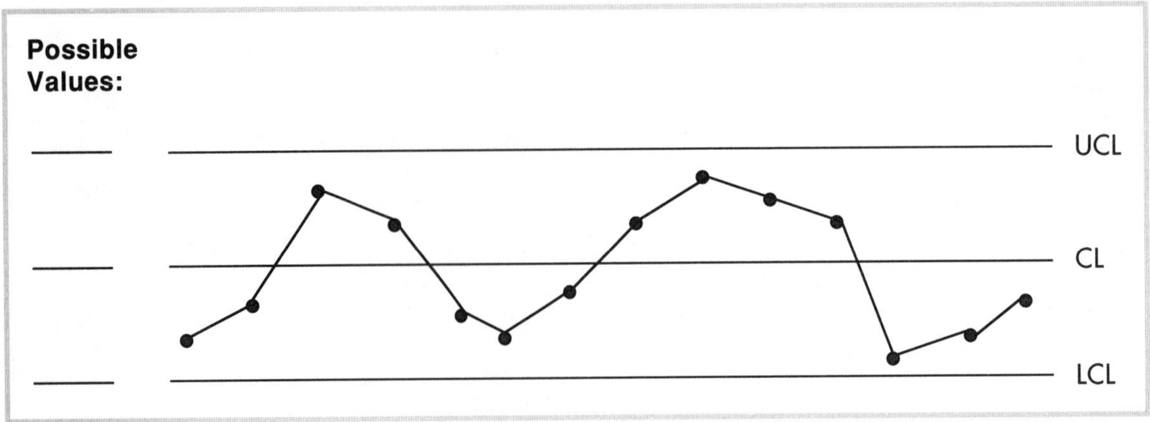

Figure 3.14.

b. Specifically, the problem with this chart is: ____________

c. This control chart could be measuring ____________

____

____

d. The following could have caused this to occur ____________

____

____

e. We would recommend taking the following actions (no action is also an appropriate option if the situation is unlikely to repeat itself): ____________

____

____

5. Figure 3.15

a. This control chart is ❑ in control *or stable* (go to next question)

❑ out-of-control *or unstable* (continue with this question)

b. Specifically, the problem with this chart is: ____________

c. This control chart could be measuring ____________

____

____

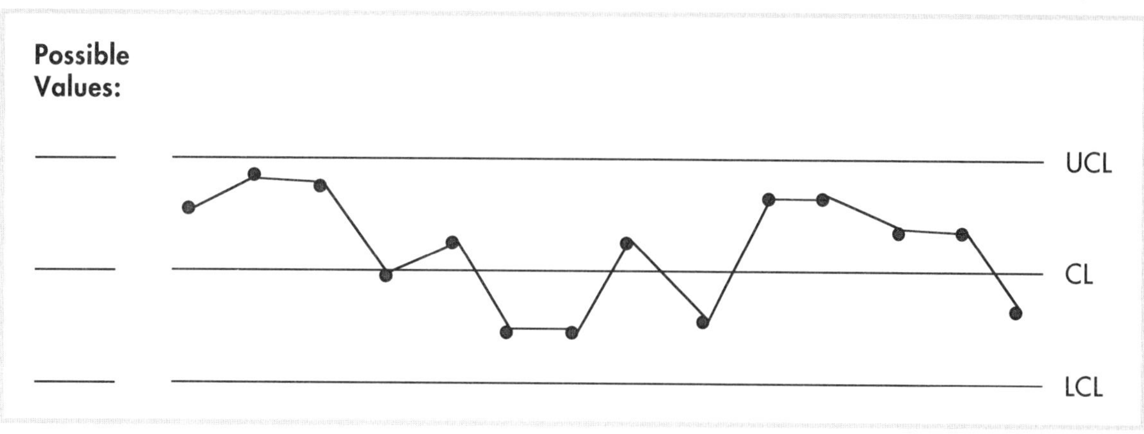

Figure 3.15.

d. The following could have caused this to occur ______________

____

____

e. We would recommend taking the following actions (no action is also an appropriate option if the situation is unlikely to repeat itself): ____

____

____

6. Figure 3.16

a. This control chart is ❑ in control *or stable* (go to next question)

❑ out-of-control *or unstable* (continue with this question)

b. Specifically, the problem with this chart is: ______________

c. This control chart could be measuring ______________

____

____

d. The following could have caused this to occur ______________

____

____

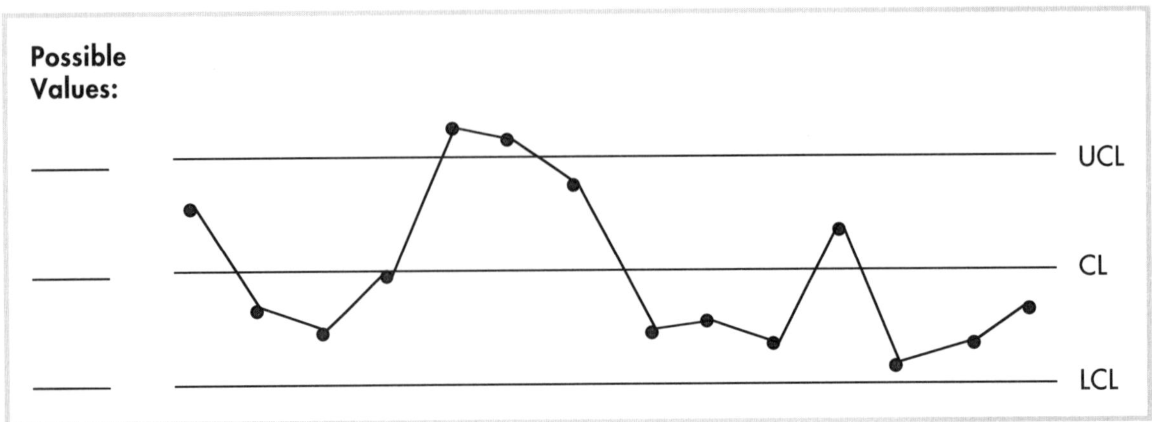

Figure 3.16.

e. We would recommend taking the following actions (no action is also an appropriate option if the situation is unlikely to repeat itself): ______________________________

____

____

References

Grant, E., and R. Leavenworth. 1980. *Statistical Quality Control.* New York: McGraw-Hill.

Mitra, A. 1993. *Fundamentals of Quality Control and Improvement.* New York: Macmillan Publishing Company.

CHAPTER 4

Choosing the Appropriate Control Chart

There are various kinds of control charts, and each has its own specific use. Until people become familiar with the different types of control charts, they generally use a flowchart or a similar device to help them choose the correct control chart for their situation. Such a flowchart is found in Figure 4.1. The flowchart is read by beginning in the center oval labeled "Start." The arrows indicate the direction of the flow, while the diamonds show the various decisions to be made. The seven rectangles at the end of each directional flow indicate the seven control charts that will be discussed briefly in this chapter. Details about calculating these charts will be covered in chapters 5 and 6.

Figure 4.1 shows that there are a total of seven widely used control charts, which are separated into two broad categories. These seven represent the most commonly used charts; however, there are other control charts available for use. The seven control charts within the two categories are attribute and variable, as follows.

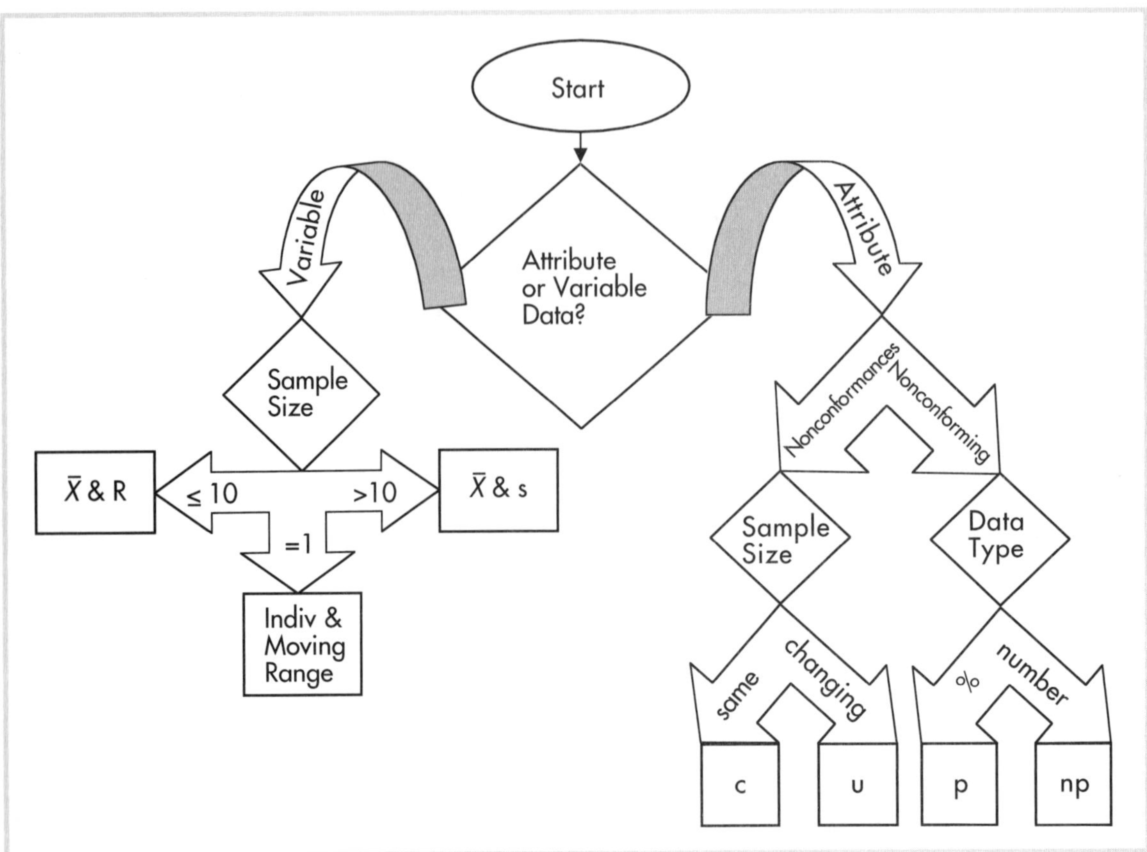

Figure 4.1. Decision flowchart for control charts.

Variable Control Charts	Attribute Control Charts
	c
$\bar{X}$ and *R*	*u*
$\bar{X}$ and *s*	*p*
Individuals and Moving Range	*np*

Attribute and Variable Data

The first decision that needs to be made is whether the data are attribute or variable. Attribute data and variable data were briefly discussed in chapter 1. It is often said that attribute data are countable while variable data are measurable. For example, we may count the number of surgical complications (attribute), but we would measure the wait time in the outpatient center (variable). Take a look at the following chart from chapter 1, and review the two types of data.

Attribute Data	Variable Data
Number of surgical complications	Wait times in the outpatient center
Number of patients in the hospital	Dollar amount of accounts receivable
Number of delinquent patient charts	Actual surgical time less scheduled surgical time

Exercise 4–1 at the end of this chapter will give you practice in determining if data are attribute or variable.

Variable Control Charts

The three variable control charts commonly used are $\overline{X}$ and R, $\overline{X}$ and s, and the individuals and moving range chart. You may have noticed from the flowchart that there are a pair of charts listed for each of the variable control chart decisions ($\overline{X}$ and R, $\overline{X}$ and s, individuals and moving range) while there are only singular charts listed for each of the attribute control chart decisions (c, u, p, and np). The reason for this is related to the primary purpose of control charts—to determine if a special cause is affecting the process. That is, we are asking if something has changed in our present process, making it different from the past process. With attribute data any of these changes will be directly reflected in the measurements. With variable data, we need to look at both the average and the variability of the data by using a pair of control charts. This concept may still be a little fuzzy to some of you—so an example will help further explain this.

A research hospital has decided to run a trial on a new drug that is thought to lower cholesterol levels. In this case we want to introduce a change (special cause) into the process to improve the treatment process—that change is the new drug. Two groups of patients agree to participate in an experiment. One group will be given the new drug, while the other will be given a placebo. Initially, every person has a cholesterol test, and an average cholesterol level is calculated for each group. By chance, the average of both groups equals 200. If the average was the only thing looked at, it would be feasible that someone would say that both groups were the same. However, one enterprising person decided to look at the variability of the data—how the individual cholesterol levels vary from each other. This person noticed that in Group 1, most of the levels were very close to 200, while the levels in Group 2 were very different from each other.

Group 1 Cholesterol Levels	Group 2 Cholesterol Levels
200	300
210	100
190	150
220	250
180	200
Group 1: Average: 200 Range: 220 − 180 = 40	Group 2: Average: 200 Range: 300 − 100 = 200

Math Refresher:

The *average* is the sum of all of the numbers divided by the number of items.

$$\text{Group 1: } \frac{200+210+190+220+180}{5} = 200$$

$$\text{Group 2: } \frac{300+100+150+250+200}{5} = 200$$

The *range* is calculated by subtracting the lowest value in the data set from the highest value in the data set.

Group 1: 220 − 180 = 40 Group 2: 300 − 100 = 200

The range is a common way to show variability. Notice that the range for Group 1 was 40 while Group 2's range was 200! Now, how similar are the groups? Obviously, they are very different, but we wouldn't have known this from the average alone—the measure of variability gave us the additional information necessary to see that the groups were really different. This same concept carries over whenever variable data are analyzed. It is rarely appropriate to look at averages only. Therefore, a control chart that shows the variability of the data (such as an *R*, *s*, or moving range chart) always accompanies an average control chart (such as an $\overline{X}$ or individuals chart).

Figure 4.2 shows the steps involved in choosing the correct variable control chart.

The next decision that needs to be made relates to the *Sample Size* diamond shown on the flowchart. When data are gathered to display on a control chart, they are chosen in subgroups or samples. The question here is how many items are in each sample. The correct control chart corresponds with the sample size, as shown in the table on the following page.

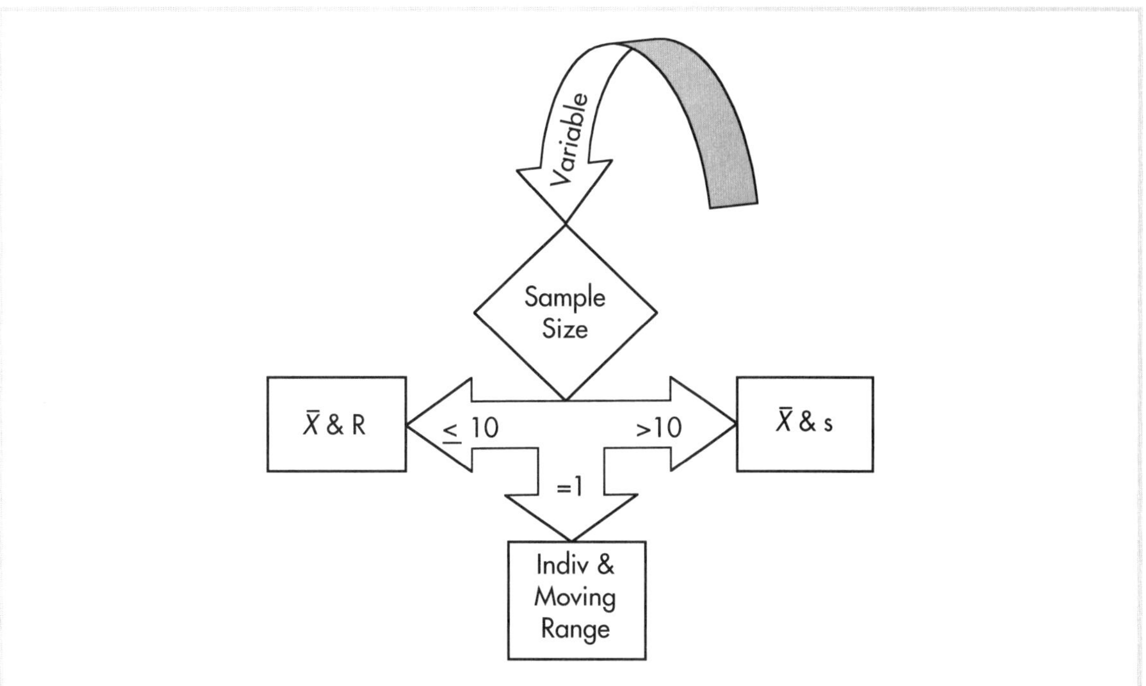

Figure 4.2. Control charts for variable data.

If the sample size is greater than 10:	$\bar{X}$ and *s* chart
If the sample size is equal to 1:	individuals and moving range chart
If the sample size is less than or equal to 10, but not 1:	$\bar{X}$ and *R* chart

The sample-size decision is one that you make ahead of time by weighing several factors that are discussed in detail in chapter 7. A brief discussion of the variable control charts follows. A detailed discussion of variable control charts with worked examples and formulas is found in chapter 6.

$\bar{X}$ and *R* Chart

$\bar{X}$ is the statistical symbol for the mean or average. Therefore, the $\bar{X}$ chart displays the averages of each of the samples. *R* is the symbol for the range. As described above, the range is the lowest value in the data set subtracted from the highest value. This is a common measure of variability that when coupled with the $\bar{X}$ chart provides a good understanding of the data set. The center line of the *R* chart is the average range, while the center line of the $\bar{X}$ chart is the overall (or grand) mean. The $\bar{X}$ and *R* chart is used with variable data when the sample size is less than or equal to 10, but not one.

> Think about something you are currently measuring that is in the form of variable data (such as weight, time, length, height, cost). When you gather data, if your sample size is greater than one or less than 11, the $\bar{X}$ and *R* chart is appropriate for your situation.

Example: A random sample of five test results is reviewed each week. The time between when the test was ordered and when the results were received are recorded and displayed on an $\bar{X}$ and *R* chart.

$\bar{X}$ and *s* Chart

The $\bar{X}$ chart displays the averages of each sample, while the *s* chart shows the sample standard deviation. The $\bar{X}$ and *s* chart is very similar to the $\bar{X}$ and *R* chart. In fact, many of the calculations are the same. The primary difference is that the s chart replaces the R chart when the sample size is larger (greater than 10). This is done because the error is smaller using the sample standard deviation rather than the range when the sample size is large. Both the range and the standard deviation give information about the variability of the data. Remember that the range is the difference between the lowest value and the highest value in the data set. In the calculation for the range, only two numbers in the data set are used (the highest and the lowest). However, the standard deviation evaluates how the values are spread out from the mean by using every value in the data set in its calculation. Like the range, the larger the standard deviation, the more variability in the data set. The standard deviation is one of the most common ways to provide information about the variability or dispersion of the data set.

Example: A random sample of 12 test results is reviewed each week. The time between when the test was ordered and when the results were received are recorded and displayed on an $\bar{X}$ and s chart. It is evident that the data type for this control chart and the previous control chart are the same. The only difference is the sample size.

> Think about something you are currently measuring that is in the form of variable data (such as weight, time, length, height, cost, and so forth). When you gather data, if your sample size is greater than 10, the $\bar{X}$ and s chart is appropriate for your situation.

Individuals and Moving Range Chart

This method is used when the sample size is one. There are frequently situations that call for this control chart. For example, a hospital may have a procedure that is performed infrequently, or is important enough that every time it is performed it should be analyzed individually. The individuals control chart displays the process average on the center line, with individual measurements plotted against the average. The moving range

> Think about something you are currently measuring that is in the form of variable data (such as weight, time, length, height, cost, and so forth). When you gather data, if your sample size is equal to one, the individuals and moving range chart is appropriate for your situation.

chart shows the variability of the data by obtaining the difference between each individual value and the previous value.

Example: A certain surgical procedure is performed approximately once per week. A study is being done to determine how much operating room (OR) time this procedure takes. Each time the procedure is performed the time is displayed individually on an individuals and moving range control chart.

Attribute Control Charts

Attribute control charts are used with attribute data. As shown in Figure 4.3, the first decision on the attribute side of the flowchart is whether we are counting the number of nonconformances on each item, or the number of nonconforming items.

This terminology comes from the original manufacturing use, but the concept is applicable to healthcare. *Nonconforming/nonconformances* means that the item does not conform to a certain standard or specification. When counting nonconformances, we are keeping track of the number of problems or items on each *thing*. For example, a medical record review might reveal that there are six different problems with one chart, and three problems with another, and so on. In those situ-

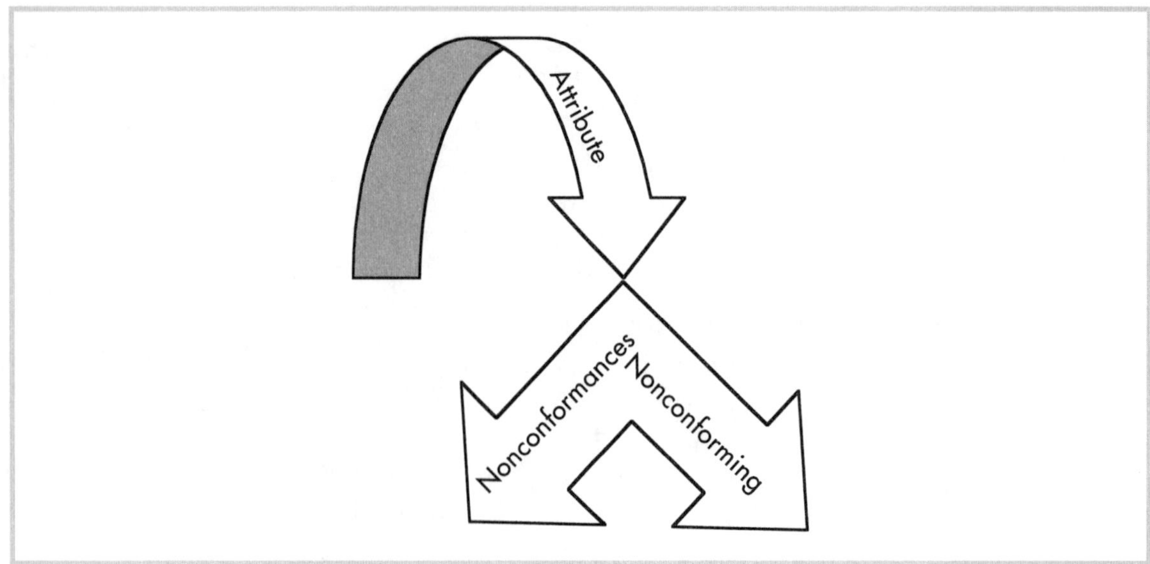

Figure 4.3. Partial flowchart for attribute data.

ations, the nonconformances side of the flowchart is appropriate because more than one problem is being counted on each item. The nonconforming side is chosen when we don't keep track of how many problems there are on each item being reviewed, we simply identify things as having a problem or not having a problem. For example, we may do another medical record review, this time looking for nothing but delinquent medical records. If a medical record is delinquent, it goes into one pile, and if it's not it goes into another. When measuring situations such as this, the nonconforming side of the flowchart should be chosen.

Nonconforming refers to recording only one thing for each item, such as whether it conforms to specifications or not.

Nonconformances refers to recording more than one thing for each item, such as the number of ways in which the item does not conform to specifications.

Examples: *Nonconforming*
The number of adverse drug reactions
The number of medication errors

Nonconformances
The number of different problems discovered on a surgical case review
The number of line items that are over-budget for each department

Although the words, nonconforming/nonconformances, have a negative connotation, they don't have to indicate an adverse situation. Initially, these words were used to measure defects/defectives. However, control charts have a much wider use than just tracking negative occurrences. Attribute control charts can also be used to display the number of occurrences of a characteristic (regardless if it is good or bad) and the number of things with one or more of the tracked characteristics. For example, we could have a control chart on the number of patients entering the emergency room (nonconforming). This chart does not measure an adverse situation for a healthcare center, nor a nonconformance with a specific standard per se. However, the chart itself may be used to determine staffing levels and patterns.

Sample/Data Decision

As shown in Figure 4.4, one of the final decisions relates to the sample itself. One of the differences between the samples for attribute and

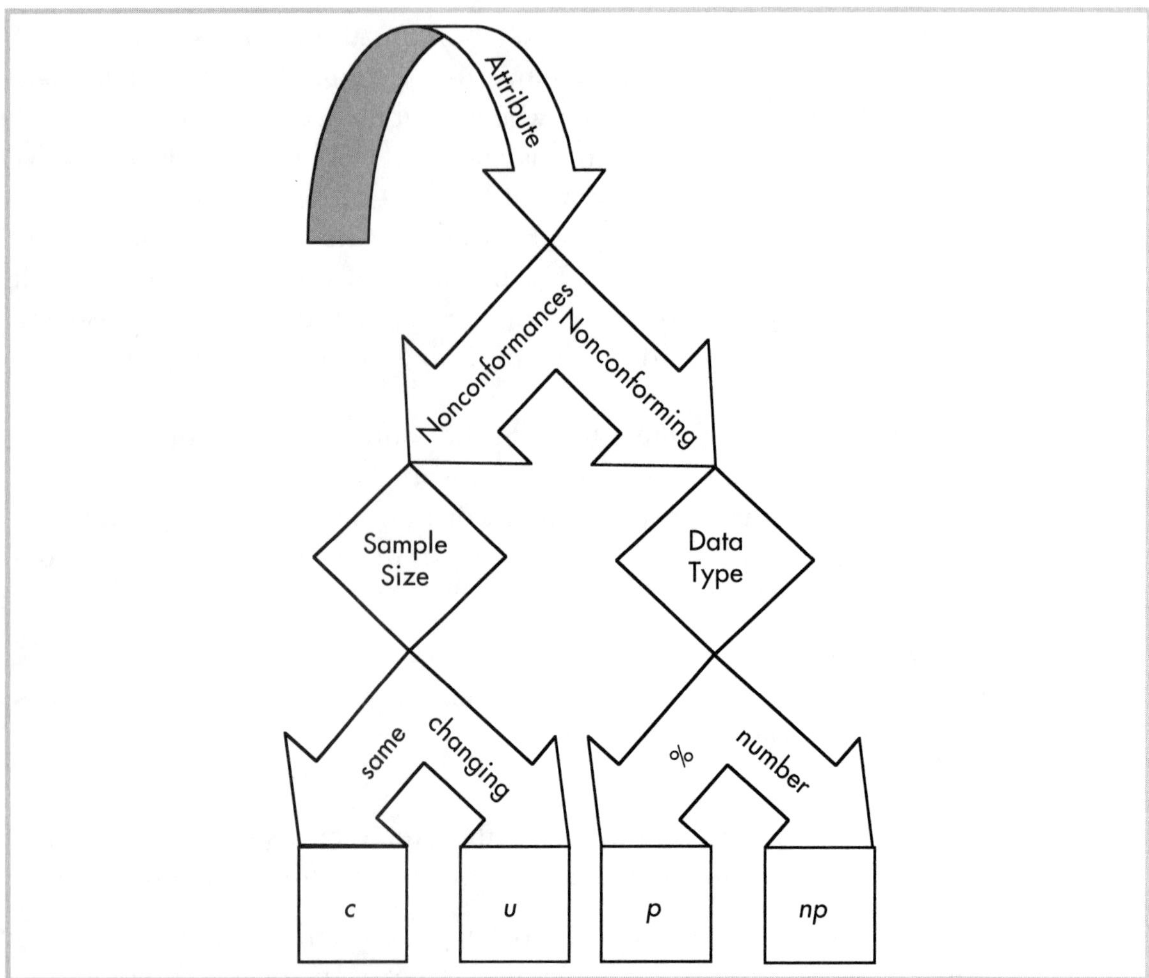

Figure 4.4. Control charts for attribute data.

variable control charts is the sample size. Sample sizes may be quite small with variable data. Attribute control charts often require larger samples because the sample must be large enough to include the problems (nonconforming/nonconformances). For example, if we know a certain problem occurs only 1 percent of the time—that's one out of 100 cases. If the sample size chosen was just 10, it would be unlikely that any problems would appear in the sample. Even a sample size of 100 or 200 may still be too small! The sample size should be consistent with the expected occurrence rate.

Another difference between the samples of attribute and variable control charts involves whether the sample size is constant or changes. Unlike variable control charts that have constant sample sizes, attribute control charts will allow the sample size to change. For example, if a manager wants to sample 5 percent of a center's daily outpatient charts, the actual sample size will change because the number of patient visits changes daily. Conversely, if a decision is made to sample 10 charts per day no matter what the actual number of visits, the sample size stays the same from day to day. The lower right side of the flowchart in Figure 4.4 identifies whether the data gathered represent a percentage or a number. Depending upon the situation, it may be appropriate to count the number of things being measured, such as the number of staff members who called in sick or to calculate the percentage, such as the percentage of staff members who called in sick.

c Chart

The *c* chart is used when tracking the number of occurrences of one or more characteristics of interest. This could include situations where nonconformances or attributes of interest for each item are being counted. This chart is based on a statistical distribution called the *Poisson distribution.* The sample size should always be equal.

Example: Every day a random sample of 20 dietary trays is chosen. A check is made between what the patient ordered and what was placed on the tray. Every incorrect item is counted for each tray.

> Think about something you are currently measuring that is in the form of attribute data (such as yes/no, under budget/over budget, right/wrong). If it is possible to count more than one thing for each item you're reviewing (nonconformances), and your sample size is a constant number, the *c* chart is appropriate for your situation.

u Chart

The *u* chart is also based on the Poisson distribution and is used in tracking the average number of characteristics of interest per item or unit examined. The *u* chart is like the *c* chart except that the sample size can change over time.

Example: Every day a random sample of 2 percent of the dietary trays is chosen. A check is made between what the patient ordered and what was placed on the tray. Every incorrect item is counted for each tray and the average number of incorrect components per tray is calculated.

> Think about something you are currently measuring that is in the form of attribute data (such as yes/no, under budget/over budget, right/wrong). If it is possible to count more than one thing for each item you're reviewing (nonconformances), and your sample size changes, the *u* chart is appropriate for your situation.

p Chart

The *p* chart is one of the most widely used attribute control charts. The *p* chart is used when tracking the percentage or proportion of the whole that is nonconforming—and each item is counted only once. The percentage is obtained by dividing the number of occurrences of a designated item by the total number of occurrences. In other words, the percentage of caesarian births may be obtained by dividing the number of caesarian births for a certain time period by the total number of births during the same time period. The *p* chart is based on the binomial distribution.

> Think about something you are currently measuring that is in the form of attribute data (such as yes/no, under budget/over budget, right/wrong). If each item being reviewed is being counted only once (nonconforming), and your data represent a percentage, the *p* chart is appropriate for your situation.

Example: The percentage of refrigerators that contain outdated medication are tracked monthly on a *p* control chart.

np Chart

The *np* chart is used when it is desirable to track the number of items that are nonconforming—and each item may be counted only once. An appropriate situation for an *np* chart is when the number of items with the characteristic is a small number within the total population under consideration. Like the *p* chart, the *np* chart is based on the binomial distribution.

Example: The number of crash carts that are missing equipment is charted monthly on an *np* control chart.

> Think about something you are currently measuring that is in the form of attribute data (such as yes/no, under budget/over budget, right/wrong). If each item being reviewed is being counted only once (nonconforming), and your data represent a number rather than a percentage, the *np* chart is appropriate for your situation.

Examples

The following examples will help you review the concepts covered in this chapter. While you read each example, think about which control chart is the appropriate one for each situation. Check your response against the explanation following each example. You will notice that many of the examples listed here cover areas that JCAHO has indicated are required measurements in the JCAHO standards.

1. You determine that you want to begin displaying your hospital's adverse anesthesia occurrences on a control chart. You decide to display the data by month. You will obtain the monthly percentage of adverse anesthesia occurrences—which is the number of adverse occurrences divided by the total number of times that anesthesia is administered each month.

   The control chart you use is a *p* chart because:

   a. You are using attribute data (yes/no for adverse anesthesia occurrence).

   b. You are measuring nonconforming data—only one thing is being measured (whether or not someone has had an adverse occurrence).

   c. You are measuring the percentage—or proportion—of people who have had an adverse occurrence (rather than the number of people).

2. You know that JCAHO requires that you measure your patients' expectations and how well you meet those expectations. From a series of focus groups you have developed a list of 10 patient expectations. You have listed these expectations on a survey that will be administered to a random sample of 20 patients per month. The patients will be asked to check *met* or *unmet* for each expectation. You will count the number of unmet expectations each month (from all 20 patients and all 10 categories), and will display this information on a control chart.

   The control chart you will use is a c chart because:

   a. You are using attribute data (met/unmet expectations).

   b. You are measuring nonconformances—more than one thing is being measured for each patient (how many expectations are unmet).

   c. Your sample size is the same for each month (20 patients).

3. You have decided to target your medication turnaround time as a performance improvement project. You decide to sample 50 records per month for the last 24 months to determine the average time it takes to administer a drug to an inpatient once the drug has been ordered by a physician. Once the control limits have been calculated using the data from the past 24 months, you plan on improving the process and want to see if there is a change as indicated by a control chart.

   The control chart you use is an $\overline{X}$ and s chart because:

   a. You have variable data (time).

   b. Your sample size is greater than 10.

4. You have a patient in your outpatient center on a weight-loss program who weighs herself once each week. The patient is very frustrated because she is interpreting the common cause variation as weight gain and/or loss each week. You want to show the patient her weight history on a control chart so she can interpret special cause as true weight losses and/or gains. You take her weekly weight from the last 30 weeks and calculate the control limits. You then ask her to plot her weight each week on the control chart so she can see when she really begins to lose and/or gain weight due to special cause rather than common cause variation.

The control chart you use is an individuals and moving range chart because:

a. You have variable data (weight).

b. Your sample size is equal to one (one person's weight is individually displayed for each week).

5. One of JCAHO's required measurements is an accounting of significant medication errors. You decide to display the data on a control chart so you can tell if you are getting better or worse over time. You gather data from the last 30 months to calculate the control limits.

   The control chart you use is an *np* chart because:

   a. You are using attribute data (yes/no for significant medication errors).

   b. You are measuring nonconforming data—only one thing is being measured (whether a significant error occurred).

   c. You are measuring the number of errors (not the percentage or proportion).

6. You have three medical-surgical floors that have similar types of patients. You want to track the average supply costs for the three floors each week to see if your overall costs are increasing, decreasing, or staying the same. In the past you have reacted whenever there has been an increase for several weeks in a row, but now you realize that you might have been overreacting to common cause variation.

   The control chart you use is an $\bar{X}$ and R chart because:

   a. You are using variable data (costs).

   b. Your sample size is less than 11 (it is comprised of the three floors).

7. You know that JCAHO has standards relating to patient restraint use. You have developed a checklist to be followed each time a restraint is used. The checklist contains five items—all of which should be checked prior to a restraint being used. As part of an improvement effort, you decide to review the last 30 months' worth of restraint use to see if all five items were covered each time a restraint was utilized. You record the number of items that were not checked prior to restraint use for each patient.

The control chart you will use is a *u* chart because:

a. You are using attribute data (met/unmet items on the restraint checklist).

b. You are measuring nonconformances—more than one thing is being measured for each patient (how many items on the checklist are unmet).

c. Your sample size varies each month (according to how many patients are in restraints for each month).

Exercise 4–2 may be used to practice choosing the correct control chart.

EXERCISE 4.1—ATTRIBUTE OR VARIABLE DATA?

INSTRUCTIONS

For each of the following examples, indicate whether the control chart should be attribute or variable. This is done by reviewing what is being measured and what type of data (attribute or variable) it involves. For example, the first item (number of delinquent medical record charts) is countable—not measurable. Therefore, the appropriate control chart is attribute.

CHART

_____ 1. Number of delinquent medical record charts.

_____ 2. Daily patient census (number of patients in the hospital).

_____ 3. Patient accounts receivable balances.

_____ 4. Patient cholesterol levels.

_____ 5. Average length of stay.

_____ 6. Scheduled appointment time less time at which patient arrived.

_____ 7. Whether or not the completed history and physical (H&P) is on the chart.

_____ 8. Patient satisfied or not.

_____ 9. Patient satisfaction level on a 1–5 scale.

_____ 10. Average age of patients on a unit.

_____ 11. Average salary level for hospital nursing staff.

_____ 12. Percent of patients with third-party insurance.

_____ 13. Time that patients wait before seeing a physician.

Think of one thing you might measure in your organization and label it attribute or variable:

_____ ____

EXERCISE 4.2—CHOOSE THE CORRECT CONTROL CHART

Review each situation below and using the flowchart in Figure 4.1, determine the appropriate control chart.

The example item (number of patients in restraints recorded by month) requires a decision of attribute or variable data. Since the number of patients is being counted (and not measured), the data are attribute. The next decision (according to the flowchart) is if nonconforming or nonconformances are being recorded. In this case, we are recording just one thing for each patient—whether or not the patient is in restraints. Therefore, the decision is to follow the nonconforming arrow of the flowchart. Finally, the last decision involves whether we are counting the number of nonconforming, or obtaining the percentage. In this case we are counting the number of nonconforming. Therefore, the appropriate chart is the *np* chart.

Example: ______ The number of patients in restraints recorded by month.

CHART

______ 1. The number of post-operative major discrepancies recorded by month.

______ 2. The average satisfaction level (from 1–5) from a patient survey given monthly to 25 patients chosen randomly.

______ 3. The percent of job interviewees who fail to keep their appointments.

______ 4. The time it takes to do a certain patient procedure that occurs rarely, and is measured each time it occurs.

______ 5. The number of repairs per unit for hospital equipment.

______ 6. The average amount of time a sample of five Registered Nurses spend on administrative tasks.

______ 7. The number of incident reports each month.

_____ 8. A 5-percent sample of employee records that are reviewed each month for four specific factors: evaluation done on time, credentials current, emergency forms in file, and training log up-to-date.

_____ 9. The time it takes to connect IV lines, recorded by patient.

_____ 10. A sample of 20 records per month to determine preadmission paperwork processing time.

CHAPTER 5

Attribute Control Charts

Overview

Chapters 5 and 6 present the calculations involved in preparing attribute and variable control charts. Generally, computer programs are used when generating control charts. These computer programs already have the formulas embedded within the software, making understanding of specific calculations optional. If the reader is planning to use control chart software and is not interested in understanding the formulas involved in generating control charts, the next two chapters may be skipped. Chapter 7 provides a brief overview of control chart software.

Attribute control charts have been defined and discussed in several places in this book already. This chapter is dedicated to the calculations involved in creating and maintaining attribute control charts. As a brief review, attribute control charts are used with data that are countable rather than measurable. Examples of attributes are yes/no, conforming/nonconforming, and problem/no problem decisions. The sample size for attribute control charts is generally larger than for variable control charts. All of the control charts in this chapter will be calculated using three standard deviations (3 sigma) for the upper and lower control limits. Discussion of other sigma levels (2 sigma, and so forth) is found in chapter 7. You will also note that while doing the calculations for the lower control limit, if a negative number is obtained, it is replaced with zero. This makes sense when you think about what is being measured. Since attributes (defects, errors, and so forth) are being measured, it is impossible to have negative values. The least number of attributes possible is zero.

In general when performing the following calculations, you may round the numbers at four digits past the decimal point. Therefore, if your calculator shows the following: 1.24386709, you would round it to: 1.2439. Most people were taught in math class that if the fifth digit is greater than or equal to 5, you round up on the fourth digit. This is generally acceptable; however, a more credible method of rounding is provided in the sidebar. After completing all of the calculations, the final answer is often rounded to two decimal places past the decimal point. Therefore, if your calculations ended with 2.4231, the final answer would be 2.42.

When using a computer program to create control charts, you may find slight discrepancies in the numbers around the third or fourth digit past the decimal point when compared to those using a calculator. This is because most computer programs do not round the numbers until the final calculation, creating a more accurate result. The difference between the hand calculations and the computer-generated numbers is called *rounding error*. An example of this is shown in the *np* calculations in this chapter. Although the hand calculations result in an upper control limit of 4.3112, the computer software package that produced the control chart in Figure 5.2 shows an upper control limit of 4.3111. The computer-generated control chart is considered more accurate.

> There are several ways to handle the rounding of numbers. The American Society of Manufacturing Engineers recommends that you retain one digit past the number of significant digits you want to end up with. Further, they recommend to round up for numbers 6–9, down for numbers 1–4, and to adopt an ongoing "rule" for 5. You decide if you will round up or down if an odd or even number follows the five. For example, you could choose to always round up if an even number follows the five and down if an odd number follows the five (or vice versa).

p Chart

A p chart is used when tracking the proportion of a population or whole and each unit is considered conforming or nonconforming. Using the example presented in chapter 4, a monthly review of refrigerators is performed to determine the percentage that contain outdated medication. In this review, all refrigerators may be targeted, or random samples of equal size may be chosen each month.

As mentioned previously, *nonconforming* refers to the lack of adherence to a standard or specified customer requirement. Let's think about the proportion of refrigerators that contain outdated medication. The standard is the date and time at which the medication is considered delinquent. Therefore, the nonconforming refrigerators are those that contain medications that don't meet the standard. The center line is calculated as follows:

Center line (CL):

$$\bar{p} = \frac{\text{Total number of nonconforming in all samples being considered}}{\text{Total number of items reviewed in all samples being considered}}$$

Although the distribution of proportions (percentages) follows the binomial distribution, we use a normal approximation of the binomial distribution to simplify calculations.

The formulas for the upper and lower control limits follow.

Upper control limit (UCL):

$$\text{UCL}p = \bar{p} + 3\sqrt{\frac{\bar{p}(1-\bar{p})}{n}}$$

Lower control limit (LCL):

$$\text{LCL}p = \bar{p} - 3\sqrt{\frac{\bar{p}(1-\bar{p})}{n}}$$

n is commonly used in statistics to designate the number of items in each sample.

A worked example will help illustrate how these formulas work. Consider that we have obtained 29 months of data from past refrigerator checks as shown in Table 5.1.

Table 5.1. Monthly Data for Outdated Medication in Refrigerators

Month	Number of Refrigerators	Number with Outdated Medication
Jan	15	3
Feb	15	2
Mar	15	4
Apr	15	1
May	15	1
Jun	15	2
Jul	15	1
Aug	15	0
Sep	15	5
Oct	15	3
Nov	15	2
Dec	15	4
Jan	15	1
Feb	15	5
Mar	15	1
Apr	15	0
May	15	3
Jun	15	3
Jul	15	2
Aug	15	1
Sep	15	2
Oct	15	2
Nov	15	1
Dec	15	6

continued

Table 5.1. continued

Month	Number of Refrigerators	Number with Outdated Medication
Jan	15	2
Feb	15	0
Mar	15	1
Apr	15	2
May	15	0
Totals	435	60

The next step is to calculate the center line.

Center Line (CL):

$$\bar{p} = \frac{60}{435} = 0.1379$$

Next, we calculate the upper and lower control limits by using the center line value calculated above (0.1379) and the number of items in each sample (15).

Upper control limit (UCL):

$$UCLp = 0.1379 + 3\sqrt{\frac{0.1379(1 - 0.1379)}{15}} = 0.4050$$

Lower control limit (LCL):

$$LCLp = 0.1379 - 3\sqrt{\frac{0.1379(1 - 0.1379)}{15}} = -0.1292 \text{ or } 0$$

The upper control limit is 0.4050 and the lower control limit is zero. The LCL is set to zero since the normal approximation gives us a negative value which is not valid for proportions. As discussed, since it is impossible in this situation to have fewer than zero nonconforming refrigerators, the lower control limit cannot be negative. The data are now displayed on the control chart as shown in Figure 5.1.

When viewing this control chart and the remaining ones in this chapter and chapter 6, keep in mind the evaluation guidelines discussed

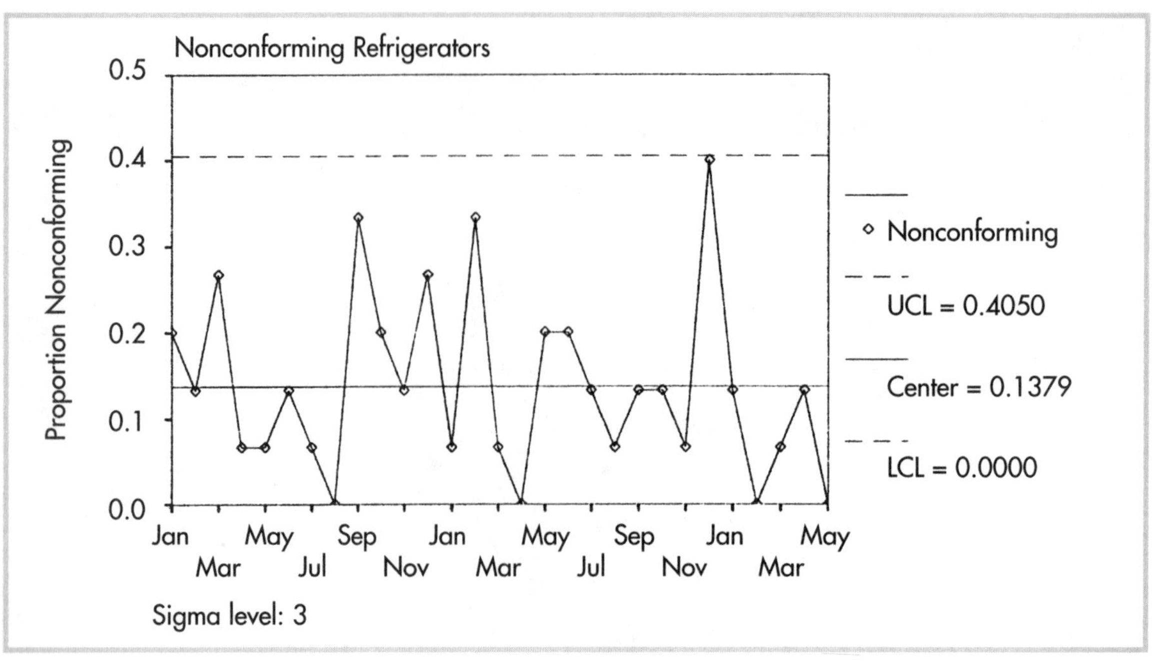

Figure 5.1. *p* chart.

in chapter 3. According to the guidelines presented, the control chart in Figure 5.1 shows a stable process. There are, however, additional guidelines by which control charts may be evaluated. They are not presented in this book, but may be found in a more advanced control chart or SPC book. A list of two recommended books is included at the end of chapter 3.

If you would like to take a few minutes to practice constructing a *p* chart, please turn to the exercise at the end of this chapter.

np Chart

The *np* chart is used when it is desirable or appropriate to track the number of items that have one or more of the characteristics of interest; for example, the number of nonconforming items. The example of an *np* chart mentioned in chapter 4 involves checking the crash carts on a monthly basis to make sure they have all of the necessary equipment. The number of carts that are nonconforming are charted on an *np* control chart. The steps involved in calculating an *np* chart follow.

Like the *p* chart, we use the normal approximation to the binomial distribution.

Center line (CL):

$$n\bar{p} = \frac{\text{Total number of nonconforming items in all samples being considered}}{\text{Total number of samples}}$$

Before the UCL and LCL are calculated, the *np* chart requires the calculation of $\bar{p}$. Since the size of each sample should be the same, $\bar{p}$ is calculated as follows:

$$\bar{p} = \frac{np}{n}$$

The formulas for the upper and lower control limits follow:

Upper control limit (UCL):

$$\text{UCL}np = n\bar{p} + 3\sqrt{n\bar{p}(1 - \bar{p})}$$

Lower control limit (LCL):

$$\text{LCL}np = n\bar{p} - 3\sqrt{n\bar{p}(1 - \bar{p})}$$

The data for the crash carts over the previous 24-month period will be used to calculate the control limits and the center line for the *np* control chart. The data appear in Table 5.2.

Since there are a total of 28 nonconforming items, and 24 samples (months), the center line is as follows:

Center line (CL):

$$n\bar{p} = \frac{28}{24} = 1.1667$$

The UCL and LCL are calculated using both $\bar{p}$ and $n\bar{p}$. As mentioned, $\bar{p}$ is calculated first. In this case, there are a total of 20 crash charts that are checked in each sample.

$$\bar{p} = \frac{1.1667}{20} = 0.0583$$

Table 5.2. Monthly Data for Crash Carts

Month	Number of Carts	Number with Missing Items
Jan	20	1
Feb	20	0
Mar	20	2
Apr	20	0
May	20	1
Jun	20	1
Jul	20	1
Aug	20	0
Sep	20	0
Oct	20	0
Nov	20	1
Dec	20	1
Jan	20	2
Feb	20	1
Mar	20	3
Apr	20	3
May	20	3
Jun	20	1
Jul	20	2
Aug	20	2
Sep	20	0
Oct	20	1
Nov	20	1
Dec	20	1
Totals	480	28

Upper control limit (UCL):

$$UCLnp = 1.1667 + 3\sqrt{1.1667(1 - 0.0583)} = 4.3112$$

Lower control limit (LCL):

$$LCLnp = 1.1667 - 3\sqrt{1.1667(1 - 0.0583)} = -1.9778 \text{ or } 0$$

The $n\bar{p}$ control chart is shown in Figure 5.2.

The control chart shown in Figure 5.2 illustrates a stable process according to the guidelines presented in chapter 3. However, if either of the next two observations (January or February) also hugs the center line (as do October, November, and December), the control chart would be considered out-of-control. The guideline it would have violated is that four of five consecutive points hug the center line. Remember, if this were to occur, there would be two immediate thoughts. It could be that someone is falsifying the data because he or she is aware of what the number *should be.* Another option is that the process has changed and the variability has been reduced. It is important to investigate the cause of this situation to know what action to take. If the process has really changed, we would want to standardize the change

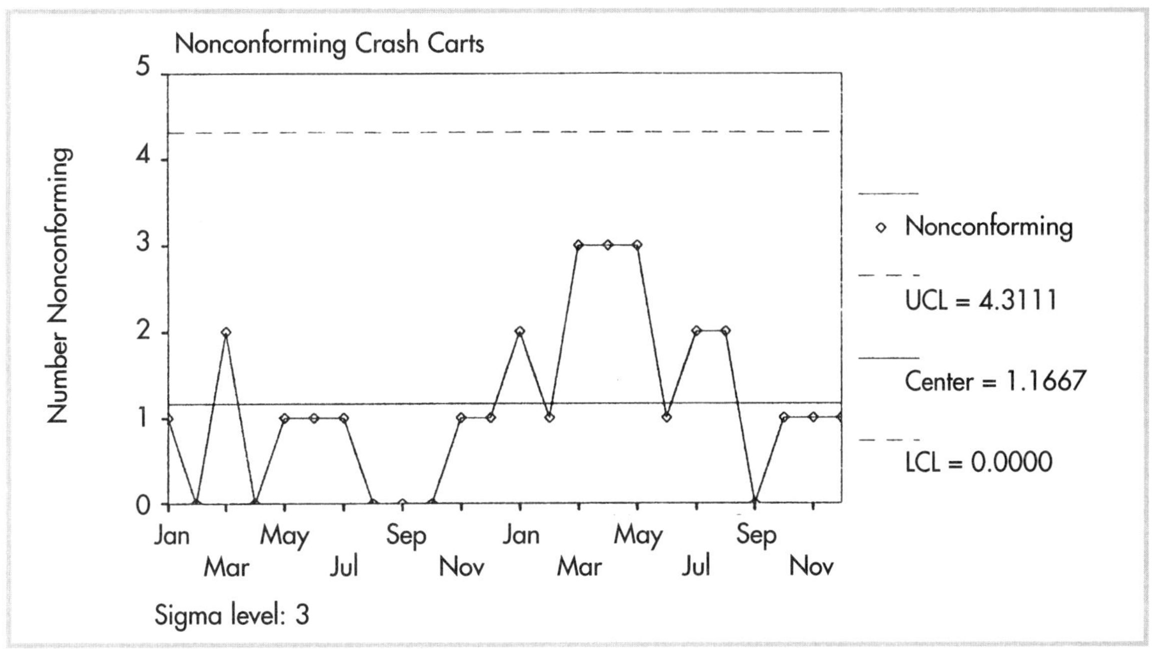

Figure 5.2. *np* chart.

(because it resulted in an improvement) and recalculate the control limits and center line.

c Chart

The *c* chart is used when tracking the number of occurrences of one or more characteristics of interest. This could include situations when nonconformances or attributes of interest for each item are being counted. The example provided in chapter 4 involved a weekly random sample of 20 dietary trays and a check between what the patient ordered and what was placed on the tray. The steps involved in calculating a *c* chart follow.

The center line is calculated by totaling the number of nonconformances, defects, or errors for each item, then dividing by the number of areas of opportunity.

Center line (CL):

$$\bar{c} = \frac{\text{Total number of nonconformances in all items sampled}}{\text{Number of the areas of opportunity}}$$

The "number of the areas of opportunity" refers to the number of clusters in which we have divided our data-gathering. This is frequently referred to as *units of time or space*. For example, if data are gathered on a weekly basis, each week becomes an area of opportunity.

Although the distribution of the number of items follows the Poisson distribution, we use a normal approximation of the binomial to simplify calculations.

The formulas for the upper and lower control limits are as follows:

Upper control limit (UCL):

$$\text{UCL}c = \bar{c} + 3\sqrt{\bar{c}}$$

Lower control limit (LCL):

$$\text{LCL}c = \bar{c} - 3\sqrt{\bar{c}}$$

In the dietary meal tray example, every incorrect item is counted for each tray and appears in the *errors* column in Table 5.3. Assume that five trays are randomly chosen and reviewed daily.

Table 5.3. Daily Dietary Error Data (Equal sample sizes)

Day	Errors	Day	Errors	Day	Errors
1	4	11	1	21	0
2	3	12	5	22	2
3	5	13	2	23	1
4	1	14	4	24	0
5	1	15	3	25	0
6	0	16	3	26	5
7	8	17	2	27	2
8	1	18	4	28	3
9	2	19	1	29	1
10	3	20	0	30	4
	Total: 28		Total: 25		Total: 18

In the table, the errors have already been totaled by column. Since the center line formula calls for the total number of errors, we simply add the three column totals together to obtain the numerator for the center line formula. In this case there were a total of 71 errors (28 + 25 + 18) over a period of 30 days. Thirty is the area of opportunity since we have chosen to group the data on a daily basis. Therefore, the center line is:

Center line (CL):

$$\bar{c} = \frac{71}{30} = 2.3667$$

In this situation, the UCL and LCL are as follows:

Upper control limit (UCL):

$$UCL_c = 2.3667 + 3\sqrt{2.3667} = 6.9819$$

Lower control limit (LCL):

$$LCL_c = 2.3667 - 3\sqrt{2.3667} = -2.2485 \text{ or } 0$$

The control chart for this example is found in Figure 5.3.

Examine the control chart in Figure 5.3 and compare the chart with the guidelines in chapter 3. You will see on the seventh day that there is a point outside of the upper control limit. This needs to be investigated because it is highly unlikely for this number of errors on dietary trays to occur unless something affected the process. For example, after investigation, we could determine that a new employee who was not properly trained started work on the seventh day. Perhaps the computerized scanner was inoperable on the seventh day. Since all patient meals are *scanned* into the system, an inoperable system would mean that each order was done manually, resulting in an increased number of errors. What should be done in these situations? Perhaps additional new-employee training is necessary, or backup procedures need to be developed for use when the computer system goes down.

Look at the points between the nineteenth day and the twenty-fifth day on Figure 5.3. You will see that there are seven consecutive points below the center line. It is unlikely for this to occur by chance. It appears likely that something happened that decreased the number of errors. In this case, we would investigate to find out what occurred. Perhaps the healthcare center's patient census was drastically decreased during this time so there was more time to make sure the dietary trays were correct. Perhaps a new procedure was tested for a period of seven days, and it resulted in a decreased number of dietary errors. If that

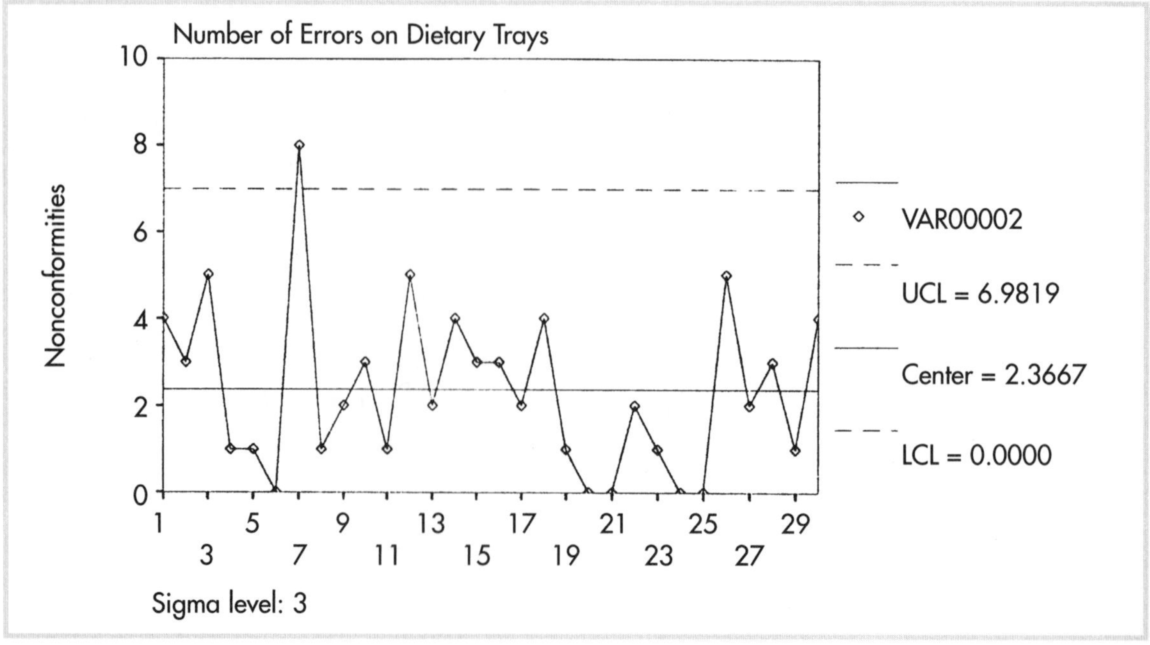

Figure 5.3. *c* chart.

were the case, we would want to standardize the change and continue to watch the process. If the improvement was sustained, we would recalculate the control limits and center line.

u Chart

The *u* control chart is used when tracking the average number of characteristics of interest per item or unit examined when the sample varies in size. Therefore, the number of nonconformances or variables of interest are counted for each item reviewed. The example provided in chapter 4 involved a daily random sample of 2 percent of the total number of dietary trays. We know that this sample size will vary because the number of patients does not stay the same from day to day. A check is made between what the patient ordered and what was placed on the tray. The steps involved in calculating a *u* chart follow.

The center line is calculated by totaling the number of nonconformances, defects, or errors for each item, then dividing by the number of items sampled.

Center line (CL):

$$\bar{u} = \frac{\text{Total number of nonconformances in all the items sampled}}{\text{Total number of items sampled}}$$

As in the *c* chart, the normal approximation to the Poisson will be used. The formulas for the upper and lower control limits are as follows:

Upper control limit (UCL):

$$\text{UCL}u_i = \bar{u} + 3\sqrt{\frac{\bar{u}}{n_i}}$$

Lower control limit (LCL):

$$\text{LCL}u_i = \bar{u} - 3\sqrt{\frac{\bar{u}}{n_i}}$$

where n_i indicates the number of items in each sample.

The upper and lower limits vary according to sample size. Instead of doing this formula once and accepting one UCL and LCL, the calculations are done each time the sample size changes.

Table 5.4 shows the data obtained using the dietary tray example with varying sample sizes.

In this example, the center line is calculated by adding up the number of nonconformances (39 + 28 = 67) and dividing that by the number of items sampled (44 + 46 = 90) as follows:

Center line (CL):

$$\bar{u} = \frac{67}{90} = 0.7444$$

The formulas for the upper and lower control limits are as follows:

Upper control limit (UCL):

$$\text{UCL}u_i = 0.7444 + 3\sqrt{\frac{0.7444}{n_i}}$$

Table 5.4. Daily Dietary Error Data (Varying sample sizes)

Day	Sample Size	Number of nonconformances	Day	Sample Size	Number of nonconformances
1	5	0	11	7	2
2	4	4	12	5	2
3	5	5	13	4	6
4	6	3	14	2	2
5	4	1	15	5	0
6	3	5	16	6	5
7	2	4	17	4	4
8	5	8	18	4	6
9	4	8	19	5	0
10	6	1	20	4	1
Totals	44	39		46	28

Lower control limit (LCL):

$$\text{LCL}u_i = 0.7444 - 3\sqrt{\frac{0.7444}{n_i}}$$

Notice that the UCL and LCL calculations are performed repeatedly instead of just once as in the previous control charts. This is because the limits change every day depending upon the sample size. Therefore, n_i (in the previous formulas) will change each time the limits are calculated, since n_i refers to the number in the sample size for each individual time frame being considered. For example, the sample size on day one was 5. Therefore, the UCL and LCL are as follows for day one:

$$\text{UCL}u_i = 0.7444 + 3\sqrt{\frac{0.7444}{5}} = 1.9019$$

$$\text{LCL}u_i = 0.7444 - 3\sqrt{\frac{0.7444}{5}} = -0.4131 \text{ or } 0$$

The control chart for this data set is shown in Figure 5.4. Notice on the figure that the UCL for day one corresponds with our calculations above (1.9019). As with the other attribute control charts, since the LCL cannot fall below zero, the calculated LCL, which is negative (–0.4131), is not used. In this situation the LCL control limit remains at zero and does not fluctuate, unlike the UCL.

Note on the chart in Figure 5.4 that the upper limit changes. This chart is evaluated in the same manner as the previous charts. In this case, there does not appear to be an out-of-control situation.

> When choosing an appropriate control chart for a given situation, there are times when aspects of a *p* chart are desired because of the reference to proportions rather than numbers; however, the sample size fluctuates as in the *u* chart. In these situations, a *p* chart for unequal sample sizes is appropriate. That chart is not introduced in this text; however, it may be found in more advanced control chart books such as the ones presented at the end of chapter 3.

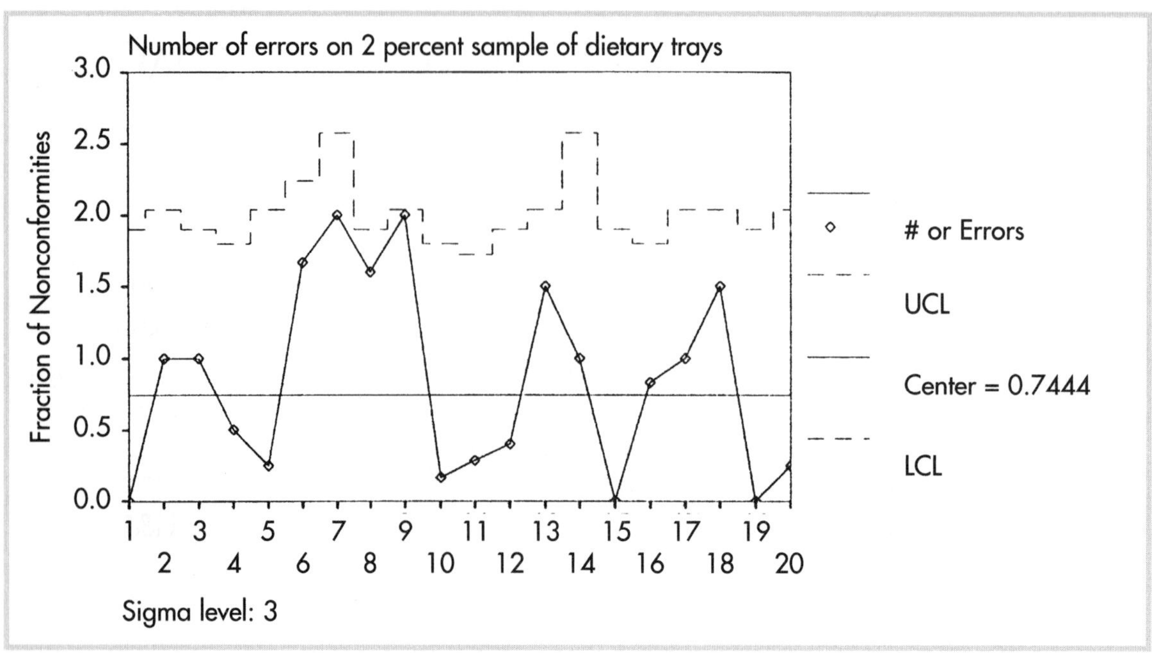

Figure 5.4. *u* chart.

EXERCISES—CREATE A *p* CHART

INSTRUCTIONS

Calculate the CL, UCL, and LCL for the *p* chart, using the data in Table 5.5. The data represent a weekly review of 10 medical records to determine if the History and Physical (H&P) is in the chart.

Table 5.5. Weekly Medical Record Data

Week	Number of Charts Reviewed	Number Missing H&P
1	10	1
2	10	1
3	10	0
4	10	2
5	10	1
6	10	0
7	10	0
8	10	3
9	10	2
10	10	1
11	10	1
12	10	0
13	10	1
14	10	5
15	10	1
16	10	0
17	10	3
18	10	2
19	10	2
20	10	1
Totals	200	27

Step 1: Calculate center line
Center line (CL):

$$\bar{p} = \frac{\text{Total number of nonconforming in all sample being considered}}{\text{Total number of items reviewed in all samples being considered}}$$

Step 2: Calculate UCL and LCL
The formulas for the upper and lower control limits follow.
Upper control limit (UCL):

$$\text{UCL}p = \bar{p} + 3\sqrt{\frac{\bar{p}(1-\bar{p})}{n}}$$

Lower control limit (LCL):

$$\text{LCL}p = \bar{p} - 3\sqrt{\frac{\bar{p}(1-\bar{p})}{n}}$$

Step 3: Draw the control chart using the following grid.

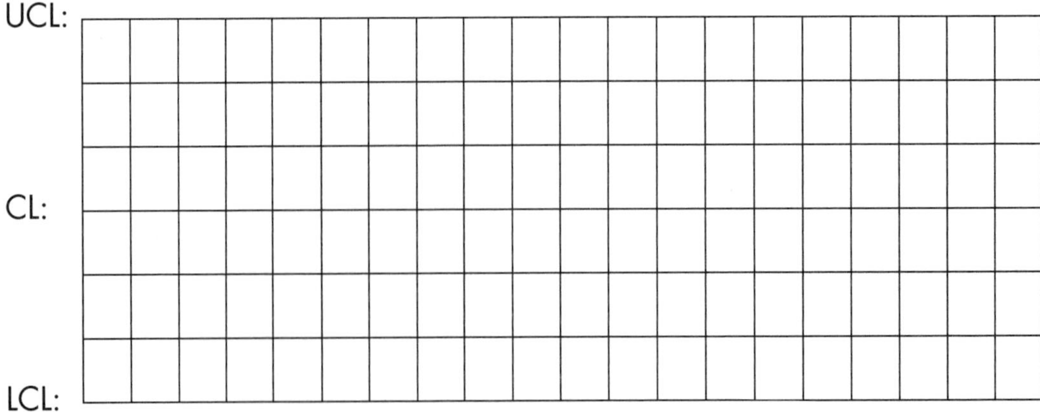

CHAPTER 6

Variable Control Charts

Overview

As mentioned in chapter 5, both chapters 5 and 6 present the calculations involved in preparing attribute and variable control charts. Most practitioners will use computer programs to generate control charts. If the reader is not interested in understanding the formulas involved in preparing control charts, chapters 5 and 6 of this book are optional, and the reader may proceed to chapter 7.

Variable control charts have been discussed previously in this book. Rather than repeating the discussion, this chapter presents the formulas involved in calculating variable control charts. As in chapter 5, all of the control charts in this chapter will be calculated using three standard deviations (3 sigma) for the upper and lower control limits. Discussion of other sigma levels (2 sigma, and so forth) is found in chapter 7. Unlike attribute control charts where negative lower limit numbers are changed to zero, the lower limits for variable control charts are presented as calculated. Another difference between the calculations of the attribute and variable control charts is that variable control charts often have formulas that call for *table values.* Table values are numbers that are obtained from a table and are based on sample size. Examples of table values used in $\bar{X}$ and R calculations that follow are A_2, D_4, and D_3. The table from which these values are obtained is found in Table 6.1.

The three variable control charts presented in this chapter are $\bar{X}$ and R, $\bar{X}$ and s, and the individuals and moving range chart.

$\bar{X}$ and R Charts

$\bar{X}$ is the statistical symbol for the mean or average and R is the symbol for the range. The $\bar{X}$ chart displays the averages of each of the samples whereas the R chart shows the variability of the data by displaying the sample range. The $\bar{X}$ and R charts are used when the data are variable and the sample size is less than or equal to 10. The example presented in chapter 4 involved a random sample of five test results reviewed weekly. The time between when the test was ordered and when the results were received are recorded and displayed on an $\bar{X}$ and R chart.

As with attribute control charts, the center line is the grand mean of the entire data set. The same is true for variable charts. For average charts we simplify the calculation of this overall average by using $\bar{\bar{X}}$. The double bar over the X indicates that this mean is a grand mean—or mean of the means. It is the overall average of all of the data.

As discussed in chapter 4, all variable control charts come in sets of two. Since we have a pair of control charts, there will be a center line for both the $\bar{X}$ and the R chart. The formula for each center line is as follows:

Center line (CL):

$$\bar{\bar{X}} = \frac{\Sigma \bar{X}}{k}$$

$$\bar{R} = \frac{\Sigma \bar{R}}{k}$$

where k is the number of samples.

There are also upper and lower control limits for both the $\bar{X}$ and the R chart. The formulas follow:

Table 6.1. Table of Constants

Sample Size	A_2	A_3	D_3	D_4	B_3	B_4	E_2
2	1.880	2.659	0	3.267	0	3.267	2.659
3	1.023	1.954	0	2.575	0	2.568	1.772
4	0.729	1.628	0	2.282	0	2.266	1.457
5	0.577	1.427	0	2.114	0	2.089	1.290
6	0.483	1.287	0	2.004	0.030	1.970	1.184
7	0.419	1.182	0.076	1.924	0.118	1.882	1.109
8	0.373	1.099	0.136	1.864	0.185	1.815	1.054
9	0.337	1.032	0.184	1.816	0.239	1.761	1.010
10	0.308	0.975	0.223	1.777	0.284	1.716	0.975
11	0.285	9.927	0.256	1.744	0.321	1.679	0.946
12	0.266	0.886	0.283	1.717	0.354	1.646	0.921
13	0.249	0.850	0.307	1.693	0.382	1.618	0.899
14	0.235	0.817	0.328	1.672	0.406	1.594	0.881
15	0.223	0.789	0.347	1.653	0.428	1.572	0.864
16	0.212	0.763	0.363	1.637	0.448	1.552	0.849
17	0.203	0.739	0.378	1.622	0.466	1.534	0.836
18	0.194	0.718	0.391	1.609	0.482	1.518	0.824
19	0.187	0.698	0.404	1.596	0.497	1.503	0.813
20	0.180	0.680	0.415	1.585	0.510	1.490	0.803

Upper control limit (UCL) $\bar{X}$ chart:

$$\text{UCL}\bar{X} = \bar{\bar{X}} + (\text{A}_2 \times \bar{R})$$

Please refer to Table 6.1 for the value of $\text{A}_{2.}$ The sample size (n) on the chart refers to the number of observations in the sample.

Lower control limit (LCL) $\bar{X}$ chart:

$$\text{LCL}\bar{X} = \bar{\bar{X}} - (\text{A}_2 \times \bar{R})$$

Upper control limit (UCL) R chart:

$$\text{UCL}R = \text{D}_4 \times \bar{R}$$

Please refer to Table 6.1 for the value of D_4.

Lower control limit (LCL) R chart:

$$\text{LCL}R = \text{D}_3 \times \bar{R}$$

Please refer to Table 6.1 for the value of D_3.

TABLE VALUES

As previously mentioned, the table values appear in Table 6.1. Another name for this table is the *Table of Constants.* You may wonder about the purpose of this table and the fact that it wasn't referred to when calculating attribute control charts. Earlier, it was stated that the control limits would be calculated using three standard deviations (3 sigma). Yet, unlike the attribute charts, you can't find a *3* or a standard deviation among them. The secret is in the tabled constants.

Worked Example

A worked example will help illustrate the use of the formulas. Consider that we have obtained 20 weeks of data from the test turnaround time review mentioned earlier. Five cases are randomly chosen each week and the time is recorded and displayed in Table 6.2. For ease of calculations in this example, the time is rounded to one-hour increments.

Table 6.2. Weekly Test Turnaround Time Data

Week	1	2	3	4	5	6	7	8	9	10
Test 1	5	4	5	1	2	4	5	3	4	5
Test 2	6	8	5	5	1	5	4	3	2	8
Test 3	6	6	8	7	5	1	3	2	3	3
Test 4	3	3	2	5	4	8	5	8	3	2
Test 5	2	6	7	5	3	2	4	6	7	9
Sum										
Mean										
Range										
Week	**11**	**12**	**13**	**14**	**15**	**16**	**17**	**18**	**19**	**20**
Test 1	4	3	5	1	7	5	4	6	6	2
Test 2	4	6	6	1	7	5	6	4	7	5
Test 3	7	5	8	8	1	2	7	6	4	8
Test 4	9	9	7	2	7	6	4	5	3	4
Test 5	3	4	6	8	4	9	5	7	3	7
Sum										
Mean										
Range										

The table format shown in Table 6.2 can actually be used to help in the calculations. The first step is to sum each week, as shown in Table 6.3. After a sum is obtained for each week, the mean is obtained by dividing the sum by the number of samples. In this case, the sum is divided by 5 and the means are shown in Table 6.3. Finally, the range is obtained by subtracting the highest number for each week from the lowest number.

Table 6.3. Completed Data for Turnaround Time

Week	1	2	3	4	5	6	7	8	9	10
Test 1	5	4	5	1	2	4	5	3	4	5
Test 2	6	8	5	5	1	5	4	3	2	8
Test 3	6	6	8	7	5	1	3	2	3	3
Test 4	3	3	2	5	4	8	5	8	3	2
Test 5	2	6	7	5	3	2	4	6	7	9
Sum	22	27	27	23	15	20	21	22	19	27
Mean	4.4	5.4	5.4	4.6	3	4	4.2	4.4	3.8	5.4
Range	4	5	6	6	4	7	2	6	5	7
Week	**11**	**12**	**13**	**14**	**15**	**16**	**17**	**18**	**19**	**20**
Test 1	4	3	5	1	7	5	4	6	6	2
Test 2	4	6	6	1	7	5	6	4	7	5
Test 3	7	5	8	8	1	2	7	6	4	8
Test 4	9	9	7	2	7	6	4	5	3	4
Test 5	3	4	6	8	4	9	5	7	3	7
Sum	27	27	32	20	26	27	26	28	23	26
Mean	5.4	5.4	6.4	4	5.2	5.4	5.2	5.6	4.6	5.2
Range	6	6	3	7	6	7	3	3	4	6

The next step is to calculate the center line for $\bar{X}$ and R. The $\bar{\bar{X}}$ formula asks us to add up the means from each week ($\Sigma\bar{X}$) and divide by the number of weeks (k). We have already calculated the means for each week in Table 6.3. When these weekly means are totaled, they equal 97.0. Since the data were gathered for 20 weeks, the center line is as follows:

Center line (CL) $\bar{X}$ chart:

$$\bar{\bar{X}} = \frac{97}{20} = 4.85$$

In order to obtain the center line for the range, all of the ranges are totaled (ΣR) and also divided by the number of weeks (k), as follows:

Center line (CL) R chart:

$$\bar{R} = \frac{103}{20} = 5.15$$

The upper and lower control limits for the $\bar{X}$ chart use a table value called A_2. A_2 is dependent upon the number of items in each sample. Since each sample (or week) contains five observations, our sample size is five. Therefore, refer to Table 6.1 and you will obtain the number 0.577. Using $\bar{\bar{X}}$, $\bar{R}$, and A_2, the formulas follow. All answers have been rounded to two digits past the decimal point.

Upper control limit (UCL) $\bar{X}$ chart:

$$\text{UCL}\bar{X} = 4.85 + (0.577 \times 5.15) = 7.82$$

Lower control limit (LCL) $\bar{X}$ chart:

$$\text{UCL}\bar{X} = 4.85 - (0.577 \times 5.15) = 1.88$$

The limits for the R Chart follow.

Upper control limit (UCL) R chart:

$$\text{UCL}R = 2.114 \times 5.15 = 10.89$$

Lower control limit (LCL) R chart:

$$LCLR = 0 \times 5.15 = 0$$

The control chart for this data set is shown in Figure 6.1.

Examine these two control charts by using the guidelines presented in chapter 3. There do not appear to be any out-of-control situations according to the guidelines. Remember, as mentioned in chapter 5, there are additional published guidelines for evaluating control charts. The basic five are the ones used in this book.

$\overline{X}$ and s Charts

As mentioned previously, when the data are variable and the sample size is greater than 10, the $\overline{X}$ and s chart is used rather than the $\overline{X}$ and R charts. The range (R) is a measure of variability that is easy to calculate and is appropriate when the sample size is small. However, when the sample increases in size, the standard deviation (s) is a better measure of variability. When the range is calculated, all of the values in the sample are ignored except for the highest and lowest value. The primary advantage of the standard deviation is that it uses all of the values in the data set to determine the variability. The example presented in chapter 4 involved a random sample of 12 test results that are reviewed each week. The time between when the test was ordered and when the results were received are recorded and displayed on an $\overline{X}$ and s chart.

The formulas for the center line and control limits follow. You will notice that the $\overline{X}$ center line formula is the same as the one presented earlier for the $\overline{X}$ and R charts.

Center line (CL):

$$\overline{\overline{X}} = \frac{\Sigma \overline{X}}{k}$$

$$\overline{s} = \frac{\Sigma s}{k}$$

where k is the number of samples.

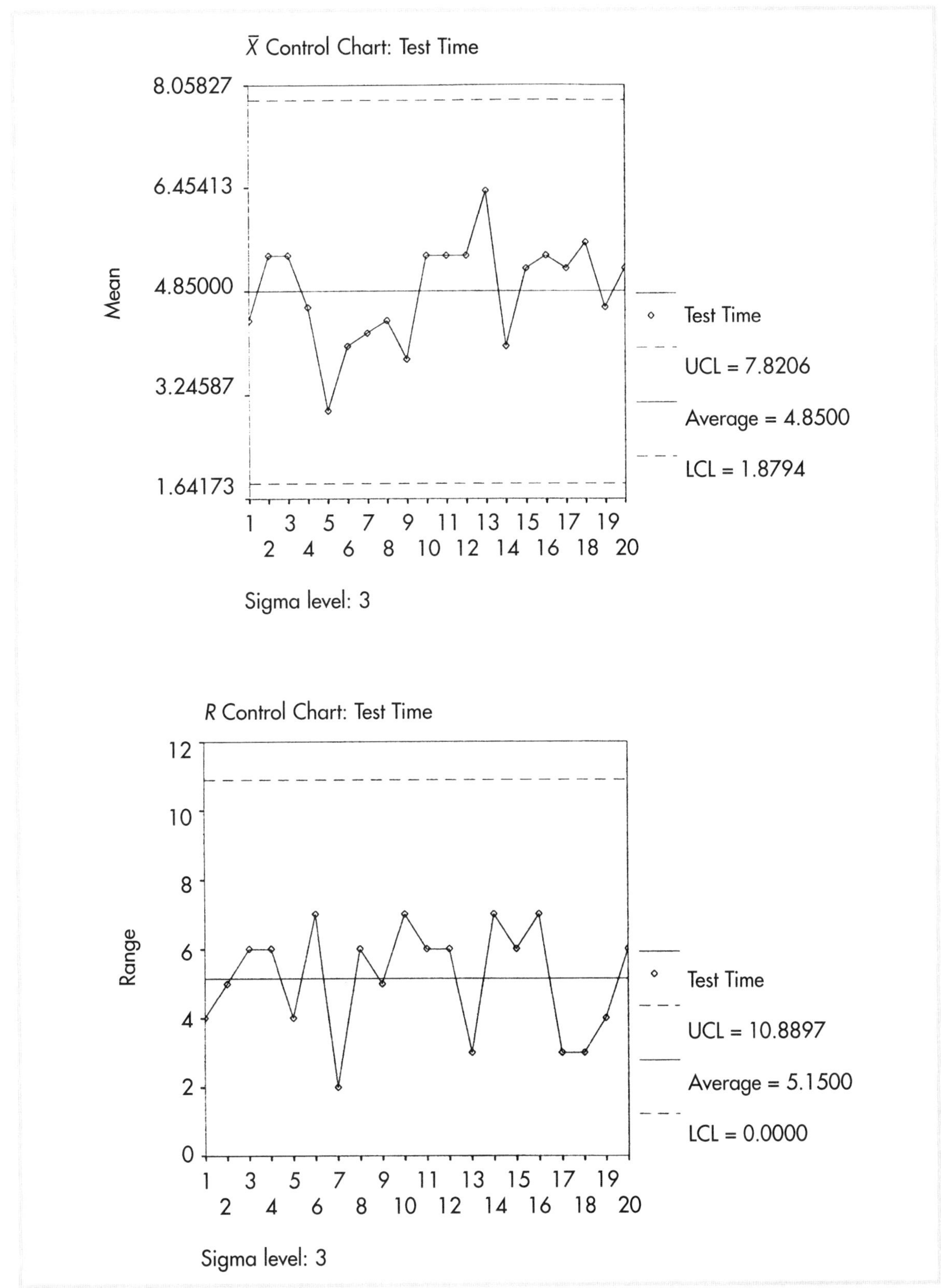

Figure 6.1. $\bar{X}$ and R control chart test times.

The upper and lower control limit formulas follow.

Upper control limit (UCL) $\bar{X}$ chart:

$$UCL\bar{X} = \bar{\bar{X}} + (A_3 \times \bar{s})$$

Please refer to Table 6.1 for the value of A_3. The sample size (n) on the table refers to the number of observations in the sample.

Lower control limit (LCL) $\bar{X}$ chart:

$$LCL\bar{X} = \bar{\bar{X}} - (A_3 \times \bar{s})$$

Upper control limit (UCL) s chart:

$$UCLs = B_4 \times \bar{s}$$

Please refer to Table 6.1 for the value of B_4.

Lower control limit (LCL) s chart:

$$LCLs = B_3 \times \bar{s}$$

Please refer to Table 6.1 for the value of B_3.

A worked example will help illustrate the use of the formulas. Consider that we have obtained 20 weeks of data from the test turnaround time review mentioned earlier. Twelve cases are randomly chosen each week and the time is recorded and displayed in Table 6.4. For ease of calculations in this example, the time is rounded to one-hour increments. As illustrated earlier in the chapter, the sum and mean are calculated for each week. In addition, the sample standard deviation is also calculated and placed on the table. There are many calculators that have standard deviation formulas preprogrammed in the calculator under the *statistics* function. There are generally two different standard deviations specified. The appropriate standard deviation is the one designated as the *sample* standard deviation rather than the *population* standard deviation. This is often indicated on a calculator with one of the following symbols:

$$\sigma_{n-1} \quad \text{or} \quad s \quad \text{or} \quad \sigma xn-1$$

It is generally not practical to calculate the standard deviation by hand. However, the formula for the hand calculation of the sample standard deviation is as follows:

$$s = \frac{\Sigma(X-\bar{X})^2}{n-1}$$

where X represents the individual values in the data set, $\bar{X}$ is the mean of the data set, and n is the number of items in the data set.

Table 6.4. Weekly Test Turnaround Time Data

Week	1	2	3	4	5	6	7	8	9	10
Test 1	4	5	3	3	3	2	3	5	4	5
Test 2	8	4	5	6	4	4	3	3	3	3
Test 3	5	4	5	8	2	4	5	3	4	5
Test 4	9	9	5	6	6	1	6	2	3	7
Test 5	6	8	5	5	7	2	7	3	3	1
Test 6	2	5	2	3	3	7	5	4	4	7
Test 7	6	6	8	7	5	7	3	2	3	3
Test 8	4	4	4	2	2	4	8	9	3	3
Test 9	8	3	2	5	4	8	5	7	3	2
Test 10	2	1	6	1	5	4	8	9	9	6
Test 11	2	6	7	5	8	2	4	6	7	9
Test 12	3	8	5	5	6	4	4	7	7	7
Sum	59	63	57	56	55	49	61	60	53	58
Mean	4.92	5.25	4.75	4.67	4.58	4.08	5.08	5.00	4.42	4.83
Standard Deviation	2.50	2.30	1.82	2.06	1.93	2.23	1.83	2.56	2.07	2.44

continued

Table 6.4. continued

Week	11	12	13	14	15	16	17	18	19	20
Test 1	4	5	5	4	4	6	8	6	6	8
Test 2	1	6	4	1	4	2	6	5	4	6
Test 3	4	3	5	6	8	5	4	6	6	6
Test 4	8	8	6	1	5	4	9	5	4	5
Test 5	4	6	6	6	5	5	6	4	7	5
Test 6	3	3	6	3	4	6	7	5	5	4
Test 7	7	5	5	5	5	3	7	6	4	8
Test 8	7	5	5	6	5	4	7	6	2	6
Test 9	9	9	7	2	5	6	4	5	3	4
Test 10	1	6	4	8	6	5	6	4	5	1
Test 11	3	7	6	8	4	9	5	1	3	7
Test 12	2	2	2	7	2	8	5	4	7	4
Sum	53	65	61	57	57	63	74	57	56	64
Mean	4.42	5.42	5.08	4.75	4.75	5.25	6.17	4.75	4.67	5.33
Standard Deviation	2.71	2.07	1.31	2.53	1.42	1.96	1.53	1.42	1.61	1.97

As presented earlier in this chapter, the table can actually be used to help in the calculations. Since the $\bar{X}$ center line calls for the *grand mean* the mean of each of the weeks are totaled and divided by the number of weeks.

Center line (CL):

$$\bar{\bar{X}} = \frac{98.17}{20} = 4.91$$

$$\bar{s} = \frac{40.27}{20} = 2.01$$

The upper and lower control limits follow.
Upper control limit (UCL) $\bar{X}$ chart:

$$UCL\bar{X} = 4.91 + (0.886 \times 2.01) = 6.69$$

Lower control limit (LCL) $\bar{X}$ chart:

$$LCL\bar{X} = 4.91 - (0.886 \times 2.01) = 3.13$$

Upper control limit (UCL) s chart:

$$UCLs = 1.646 \times 2.01 = 3.31$$

Lower control limit (LCL) s chart:

$$LCLs = 0.354 \times 2.01 = 0.71$$

The $\bar{X}$ and s control chart is shown in Figure 6.2.

After a review of Figure 6.2, and a comparison with the guidelines listed in chapter 3, it appears that there are no out-of-control situations.

Individuals and Moving Range Chart

There are times when it is not possible, too expensive, or impractical to gather data in samples. In these situations data are gathered and tracked individually. When this occurs we say that $n = 1$, or the sample size is equal to one. Each individual value is displayed on the individuals (or X) chart, while the differences between consecutive values are tracked on the moving range chart. The example in chapter 4 involves a certain surgical procedure that is performed approximately once per week. A study is being done to determine how much operating room (OR) time this procedure takes. Each time the procedure is performed, the time is displayed individually on an individuals and moving range control chart.

The center line and control limit formulas follow.

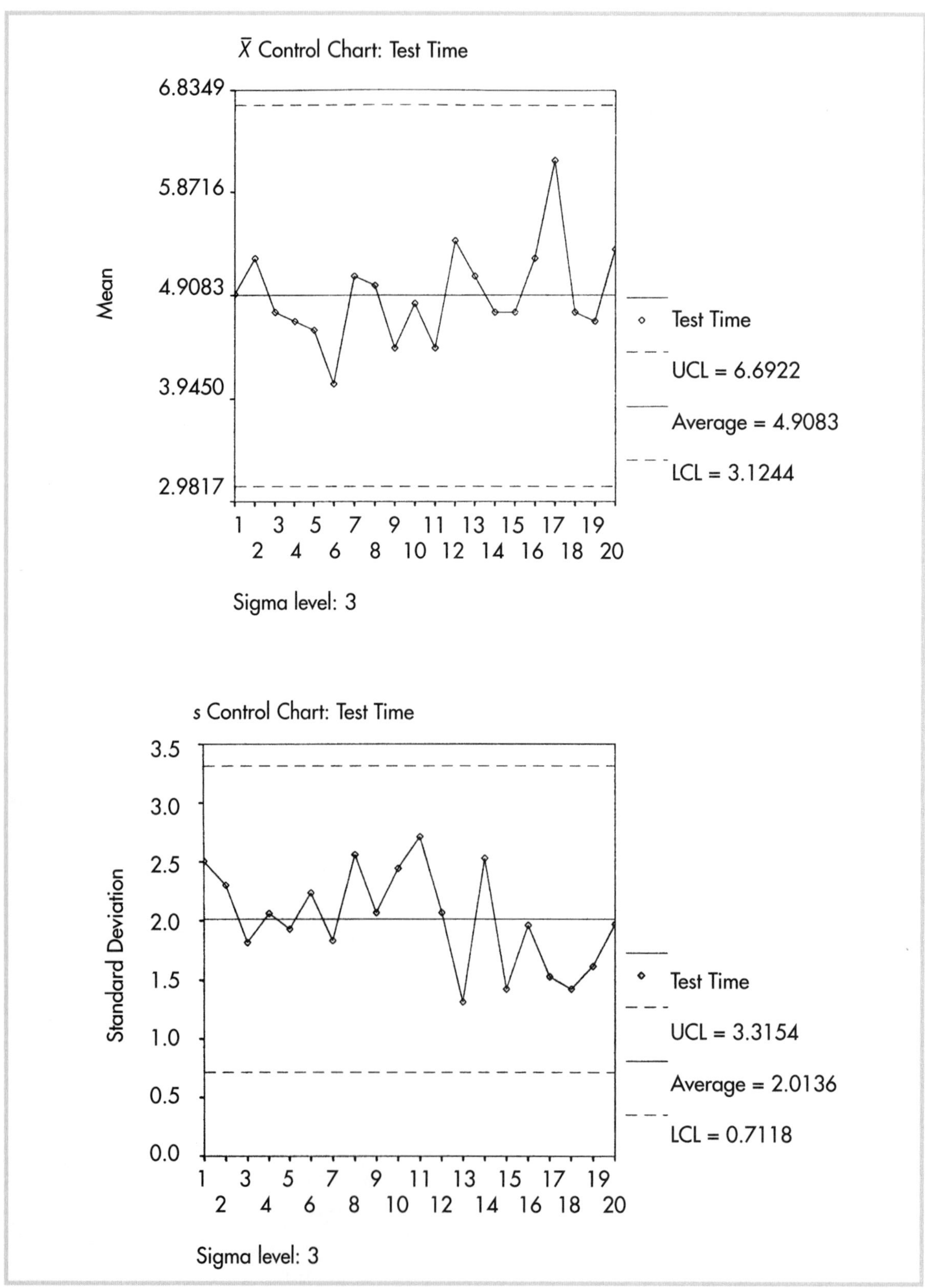

Figure 6.2. $\bar{X}$ and s control chart test times.

Center line (CL):

$$\bar{X} = \frac{\Sigma X}{k}$$

$$\overline{MR} = \frac{\Sigma MR}{k - 1}$$

where k is the number of samples.

The upper and lower control limit formulas follow.

Upper control limit (UCL) $\bar{X}$ chart:

$$\text{UCL}X = \bar{X} + (\text{E}_2 \times \overline{MR})$$

Please refer to Table 6.1 for the value of E_2. The sample size (n) on the chart refers to the number of observations used in the moving range calculations.

Lower control limit (LCL) $\bar{X}$ chart:

$$\text{LCL}X = \bar{X} - (\text{E}_2 \times \overline{MR})$$

Upper control limit (UCL) moving range (MR) chart:

$$\text{UCL}MR = \text{D}_4 \times \overline{MR}$$

Please refer to Table 6.1 for the value of D_4, using a sample of size 2 since each range is based on only two readings.

Lower control limit (LCL) moving range (MR) chart:

$$\text{LCL}MR = \text{D}_3 \times \overline{MR}$$

Please refer to Table 6.1 for the value of D_3 using a sample of size 2.

Using the example given in chapter 4 and mentioned previously, the times (by minute) for the surgical procedure being tracked are given in Table 6.5.

The calculations for the control chart follow.

Center line (CL):

Table 6.5. Surgical Procedure Time Data

Procedure Occurrence	Time in Minutes
1	128
2	123
3	173
4	201
5	136
6	181
7	152
8	155
9	170
10	103
11	130
12	106
13	128
14	183
15	152
16	160
17	138
18	153
19	158
20	142
21	147
22	120
23	142
24	186
25	110
Total	3677

$$\bar{X} = \frac{3677}{25} = 147.08$$

In order to obtain the moving range, the time value for each procedure is subtracted from the following procedure, and the positive value is presented. For example, the time for Procedure 1 is 128. Therefore, 128 is then subtracted from the time for Procedure 2 (123), as follows:

$$123 - 128 = -5$$

Since the range is always presented as a positive value, the range becomes 5. Therefore, the moving range is 5 as shown in the *Moving Range* column under Procedure 2 in Table 6.6.

Center line (CL):

$$\overline{MR} = \frac{706}{25 - 1} = 29.42$$

The upper and lower control limit formulas follow. The value for E_2 is obtained by determining the number of observations used in the moving range calculations. Since two observations were used in this case (the moving range is obtained by subtracting each value from its successive value), $n = 2$, making E_2 equal to 2.659. D_4 and D_3 are obtained in a similar manner.

Upper control limit (UCL) *X* chart:

$$UCLX = 147.08 + (2.659 \times 29.42) = 225.29$$

Lower control limit (LCL) *X* chart:

$$LCLX = 147.08 - (2.659 \times 29.42) = 68.87$$

Upper control limit (UCL) moving range (*MR*) chart:

$$UCLMR = 3.267 \times 29.42 = 96.11$$

Table 6.6. Surgical Procedure Time Data with Moving Range

Procedure Occurrence	Time in Minutes	Moving Range
1	128	
2	123	5
3	173	50
4	201	28
5	136	65
6	181	45
7	152	29
8	155	3
9	170	15
10	103	67
11	130	27
12	106	24
13	128	22
14	183	55
15	152	31
16	160	8
17	138	22
18	153	15
19	158	5
20	142	16
21	147	5
22	120	27
23	142	22
24	186	44
25	110	76
Total		706

Lower control limit (LCL) moving range (*MR*) chart:

$$\text{LCL}MR = 0 \times 29.42 = 0$$

The individuals and moving range chart is shown in Figure 6.3. The individuals chart shows many of the data points hugging the center line during weeks 15 to 23. It is possible that the process has reduced its variability due to a special cause. When examining the moving range chart, at least seven consecutive points are below the center line during approximately the same time frame. The reasons for these occurrences should be explored. If, in fact, the special cause is an improvement in the process that may be standardized, this should be done. It may then be possible to recalculate the control limits, assuming the decreased variability is sustained.

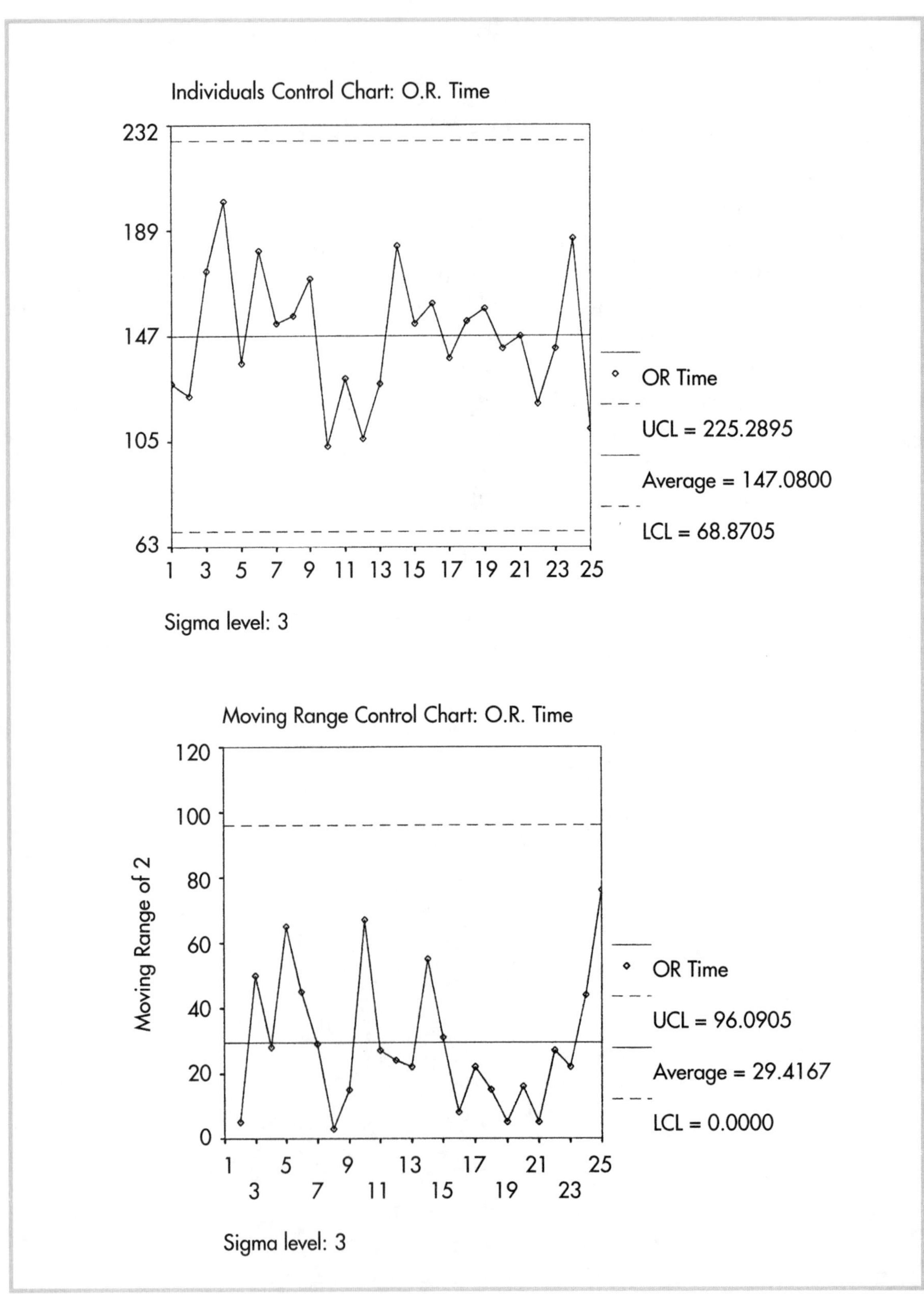

Figure 6.3. Individuals and moving range control charts.

EXERCISES—CREATE AN $\bar{X}$ AND R CHART

INSTRUCTIONS

Calculate the CL, UCL, and LCL for the $\bar{X}$ and R chart, using the data in Table 6.7. The data represent a weekly review of five records to determine the time that patients wait until seeing a physician in the outpatient center.

Step 1: Complete Table 6.7 to assist in calculating the center lines for the $\bar{X}$ and R charts:

Center line (CL):

$$\bar{\bar{X}} = \frac{\Sigma \bar{X}}{k}$$

$$\bar{R} = \frac{\Sigma R}{k}$$

where k is the number of samples.

Step 2: Calculate UCL and LCL for the $\bar{X}$ chart:

The formulas for the upper and lower control limits follow.

Upper control limit (UCL) $\bar{X}$ chart:

$$\mathrm{UCL}\bar{X} = \bar{\bar{X}} + (A_2 \times \bar{R})$$

Please refer to Table 6.1 for the value of A_2. The sample size (n) on the chart refers to the number of observations in the sample.

Lower control limit (LCL) $\bar{X}$ chart:

$$\mathrm{LCL}\bar{X} = \bar{\bar{X}} - (A_2 \times \bar{R})$$

Table 6.7.

Week	1	2	3	4	5	6	7	8	9	10
Test 1	15	24	5	12	35	10	25	15	15	32
Test 2	5	23	15	42	10	20	45	19	12	18
Test 3	35	30	25	28	24	15	30	23	29	10
Test 4	21	15	33	10	19	25	15	41	20	35
Test 5	23	10	34	26	20	25	34	38	10	42
Sum										
Mean										
Range										

Week	11	12	13	14	15	16	17	18	19	20
Test 1	14	13	25	31	18	45	14	26	36	22
Test 2	12	32	12	42	20	25	23	42	11	3
Test 3	31	34	26	28	12	13	18	19	39	31
Test 4	30	15	13	12	25	18	25	28	24	20
Test 5	24	25	18	17	32	35	29	35	22	5
Sum										
Mean										
Range										

Step 3: Calculate UCL and LCL for the *R* chart:
Upper control limit (UCL) *R* chart:

$$\text{UCL}R = \text{D}_4 \times \bar{R}$$

Please refer to Table 6.1 for the value of D_4.
Lower control limit (LCL) *R* Chart:

$$\text{LCL}R = \text{D}_3 \times \bar{R}$$

Please refer to Table 6.1 for the value of D_3.

Step 4: Draw the control chart on the grid below.

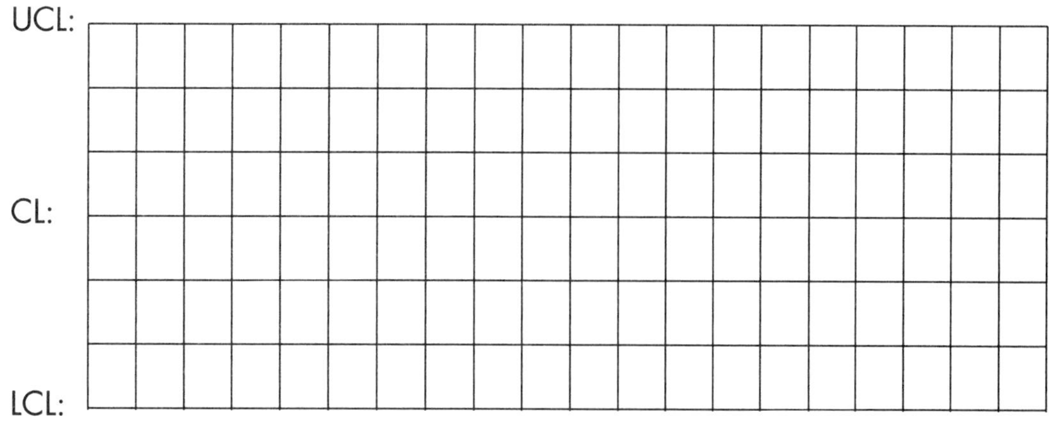

CHAPTER 7

Beginning to Use Control Charts

There are some general steps involved in the use of control charts. The steps are outlined, and a discussion follows.

Steps in Using Control Charts

1. Select the characteristic to be measured.
2. Determine the sample size and sampling frequency.
3. Determine the appropriate control chart.
4. Gather and record data.
5. Calculate the center line and control limits.
6. Review the control chart and revise control limits if necessary.
7. Implement and monitor the control chart.

Step 1: Select the Characteristic to be Measured

There are several things to be considered when determining what will be measured. One consideration is to choose characteristics that are key to the primary purpose of the organization. Leadership should be well aware of these items, but in addition, reference to these key items will most likely appear in the strategic plan and PI Plan. The time and cost involved in gathering the data will also impact what data will be measured. In addition, required regulatory items must be measured as well as problem-prone, high-risk, or high-volume procedures. Finally, we want to make sure that the item being measured is appropriate and will provide us with the desired information about the performance of the process being considered. These considerations should be weighed together when determining exactly what will be measured. Sometimes organizations have the problem of having too many items to measure. When this is the case, a selection grid may be helpful to determine which variable(s) to measure. An example of a selection grid is shown in Table 7.1.

The selection grid is used by listing possible variables for measurement along the top row. Each variable is then evaluated by assigning point values in response to the questions listed along the first column. The individuals using the grid may determine the point value ranges.

Table 7.1. Selection Grid

	Variable #1	Variable #2	Variable #3	Variable #4
Is variable part of a key organizational process?				
Is variable part of a high-risk procedure?				
Is variable part of a high-volume procedure?				
Is variable part of a problem-prone area?				
Are data inexpensive to gather?				
Are data non-time consuming to gather?				
Is there potential for improvement?				

The value range may also be different for each row. For example, if an organization wanted to give more emphasis to variables relating to key organizational factors, the range of possible values in this area may be greater (that is, 0–5) than for high cost variables (that is, 0–2). After completing the grid, the columns are totaled. The column with the highest total may be the first variable to be measured. An example of a completed grid is found in Table 7.2.

The variable scoring the highest (variable #3 at 9) is the one that should be measured prior to the other two variables, according to the selection grid. Once the characteristic is determined, the data type plays a key role in the control chart. The data will be attribute (countable, yes/no) or variable (measurable, numeric). Occasionally data may be both. For example, on-time status may be measured as an attribute with late/on-time as the only two options, or as variable data with the actual minutes recorded. In situations where both may be used, it is generally preferable to choose to gather the variable data unless it is cost-prohibitive to do so. This is true because ultimately the variable data may be converted to the attribute data, but the reverse is not true. For example, if time is the information being gathered, a later

Table 7.2. Completed Selection Grid

	Variable #1	Variable #2	Variable #3
Is variable part of a key organizational process?	2	1	2
Is variable part of a high-risk procedure?	1	1	2
Is variable part of a high-volume procedure?	0	2	2
Is variable part of a problem-prone area?	0	0	0
Are data inexpensive to gather?	2	1	1
Are data non-time consuming to gather?	0	1	1
Is there a good potential for improvement?	1	2	1
Total	6	8	9

Point Values: 0–No; 1–Somewhat; 2–Yes.

determination may be made as to a late/on-time status. However, if only late/on-time information is gathered, the time designation may not be derived from these attribute data. Consequently, if further data analysis is desired in the future, the variable data offer more possibilities than the attribute data.

Step 2: Determine the Sample Size and Sampling Frequency

How many measurements should be taken for each sample and how should sampling take place? Unfortunately, the answer is "enough." The number of samples depends on the process and the expected effect of special causes. One consideration is that some control charts require that the sample sizes are equal—in other words, each time we gather data, we look at the same number of items.

Initially, control charts are often used in existing situations where data have been collected in the past, and the control chart is being used as a new way to display and analyze the data. In many cases, it is possible to continue with the existing sample size to see how it works within the control chart. Changes to the sample size may be made later after a more thorough understanding of the process and its common and special causes, and after the control chart itself is obtained. This also applies to the frequency of sampling. Obviously, the more frequently the samples are drawn, the more time-consuming and costly the process. However, it is possible to miss important information by using only infrequently drawn samples.

Ideally you would want to sample only when special causes occur. This would be the most efficient and effective sampling method. It is also impossible unless you are clairvoyant. So, you may want to begin with frequent sampling to better understand the process and to catch and correct problems as they occur. Once many of the problems have been addressed, it may be possible to reduce the sampling size and/or frequency.

The primary sampling considerations are often different for attribute and variable control charts. A discussion of the guidelines for each follows.

VARIABLE CONTROL CHART SAMPLING CONSIDERATIONS

Shewhart, the original inventor of control charts, suggested that the sample size of four is appropriate for many situations using variable data. In the manufacturing setting, a sample size of five is frequently used. The initial reason for this is when control charts were originally introduced, many workers had poor arithmetical skills and the personal calculator was not yet invented. To make it easy to perform the calculations, sample sizes of five or 10 were used. Now the use of the sample size five or 10 is bound in "tradition."

Individuals control charts (sample size = 1) are used when the cost of sampling is very high or when only one measurement is available or appropriate (for example, if the process has very little inherent variability or if taking a measurement will affect the process for a period of time). Larger samples may be used when we want a control chart that is very sensitive to small special cause variations. As the sample size increases, the upper and lower control limits move closer to the center line, increasing the *sensitivity* of the control chart.

Another name for the samples used in control charts is *subgroups.* A great deal has been written about the subject of *rational subgroups.* or *rational samples.* This involves the decision in determining the sample size and when to sample. A brief summary of some of the primary issues in determining rational samples follows.

The upper and lower control limits on the $\bar{X}$ control charts are based on the variability of the data within the samples. For this reason, we want to determine samples that make sense—or are rational. There are two general rules to be considered when determining rational samples. The samples should be homogeneous *within* themselves, and the variation *between* the samples should be appropriate to determining the limits on the normal variation between the samples. By *homogeneous,* we mean that the data values within each sample should be similar to each other. Another way of looking at this is that all the variation within a sample should be due to common cause variation, with little chance of special cause variation. For example, three readings of the pulse level of an individual should be similar to each other during daytime hours. If we intermix a "resting" pulse level within this group of daytime pulse levels, the sample is no longer homogeneous.

In order to determine if the variation between the samples is appropriate, identification of the sources of variation should be completed. Personal discretion coupled with an understanding of the process will help in determining a rational sample.

Attribute Control Chart Sampling Considerations

The primary difference between the samples for attribute and variable control charts is the sample size. Sample sizes may be quite small with variable data. Attribute control charts often require larger samples—sometimes in the hundreds. The larger sample sizes are often necessary when the nonconforming attribute occurs infrequently; therefore, many observations must be taken in order to obtain any nonconforming data in the sample.

Step 3: Determine the Appropriate Control Chart

Chapter 4 contains detailed instructions on choosing the appropriate control chart for various data types and sample sizes. Use the flowchart provided in chapter 4 to determine the appropriate control chart for your measurement situation.

Step 4: Gather and Record Data

There are many opportunities for bias to enter the measurement within the data gathering efforts. Some of the considerations that take place in the data gathering process are as follows:

Unbiased sampling techniques

Reliability

Validity

Timeliness

Unbiased Sampling Techniques

Whenever possible, data should be gathered using random sampling techniques. The four most common random sampling techniques are:

Simple random sampling

Stratified random sampling

Systematic sampling

Cluster sampling

Some of these methods have been briefly mentioned in chapter 1 of this book. Further instruction on random sampling techniques is available in statistics textbooks. The advantage of random sampling techniques is that they take the sample decision making away from individuals. Even though people usually think they are choosing a fair and unbiased sample, it often is not the case. The use of a random technique helps eliminate a certain bias called *selection bias.* Selection bias occurs when the items selected to be in the sample are in some way different from the items not selected to be in the sample.

Reliability and Validity

Reliability relates to consistency in the measurement, while *validity* relates to the confidence that we have in the inferences we can make from the data because we have measured what we are intending to measure. *Reliable data* are data that are gathered the same way each time. For example, if four different nurses are gathering data in four different ways, they will probably end up with data that are very unreliable. *Valid data* are data that are actually measuring what we think we are measuring. For example, if a monitor is not working properly, we may think that we're gathering a certain type of data, when in fact, the data are really a reflection of the malfunctioning unit, making our data invalid.

In many cases, the reliability and validity of the measurement may be increased by using a check sheet accompanied by an operational definition. A *check sheet* is generally a piece of paper that has a grid on it with designations of various categories of interest. The data collector

	Day 1	Day 2	Day 3
Patient one minute late or more	///	/	/
Medical record not pulled	////	///	////

Figure 7.1. Check sheet reasons for clinic delays.

uses the check sheet to record the frequency of each occurrence of the various categories as listed on the check sheet. An example of a partially completed check sheet is shown in Figure 7.1. This check sheet was used to gather data to determine the frequencies of occurrences that caused the clinic to experience delays. A further explanation of check sheets is provided in chapter 8.

Another tool that will help eliminate bias in data gathering is an *operational definition.* An operational definition is a written statement that provides information and instructions to the data collector(s) regarding the data to be gathered. This is important because people often have different interpretations of even general statements. The need for an operational definition was clear when a particular surgical unit decided to gather data on the scheduled time of surgeries versus the actual time the surgeries began. In this situation members of the surgical nursing staff were asked to record the time surgeries started for a period of one week. When the data were compiled, it was clear that there were some discrepancies. The nurses were called together to discuss how they gathered the data. It turned out that each nurse defined *surgery began* differently. It was agreed that the following week the data collected would reflect the time at which the first incision was made. Further explanation of an operational definition is found in chapter 8.

TIMELINESS

Just like a loaf of day-old bread, the value of data is reduced as time goes on. Some organizations gather data, wait until there's enough accumulated to enter into the computer, send the data to someone to enter, get the results, and set them on the shelf until a meeting is held to review the data. Six months can pass while all of this takes place. By that time the data are like moldy loaves of bread—no good anymore! It is important to gather timely data and then use data as soon as possible.

Step 5: Calculate the Center Line and Control Limits

The formulas for calculating the center line and control limits for the seven most commonly used control charts are found in chapters 5 and 6. Many organizations choose to purchase computer software to perform the calculations rather than doing the calculations by hand. There are many software packages available and most are fairly inexpensive and easy to use. Some of these packages have Web sites that allow the prospective user to download a sample of the software package to test before purchasing. Although the author does not specifically endorse any of the packages, a list of some of the packages available is found in Table 7.3.

Most computer control chart packages operate in a similar manner. The user will generally enter (or import) data on a screen that has a series of rows and columns. Once the data are entered and saved, the user will choose the appropriate control chart. This step assumes that the user knows which control chart to choose. The computer will perform the calculations regardless of the appropriateness of the control chart chosen, as the software has no way of knowing if

Table 7.3. Control Chart Software

Name	Phone	Web Site
JMP (SAS Institute)	919-677-8000	www.JMPdiscovery.com
PFT Professional	1-800-870-4200	www.lqd@iqd.com
QI Analyst (SPSS Inc.)	1-800-321-3623	www.spss.com/software/quality/
SQCpack	1-800-777-3020	www.pqsystems.com
Statistica	918-749-1119	www.statsoft.com

the correct control chart has been designated. Therefore, it is important that the user understands the assumptions behind each of the control charts, and chooses the correct one. There are some control chart packages that lead the user through a series of prompts that help determine the correct control chart; however, most do not. Once the user designates the control chart, the computer completes the calculations and presents a visual display of the control chart. The user may continue to add data to the original file and create and print updated control charts as time goes on.

Determining Control Limit Sigma Levels

Whether you will be performing hand calculations or using statistical control chart software, one of the decisions that may be made is how many sigma levels will be used. The default value on control chart software (as well as the formulas for hand-calculations) is 3-sigma, which means that the control limits are set three standard deviations above and below the center line. This is the most common sigma level, and is the one to be used unless specific circumstances dictate a different sigma level. An understanding of how the standard deviations function will help in understanding this topic.

The control limits of a control chart are probability limits that are based on specific statistical distributions. A 3-sigma limit indicates that the probability of a point falling above the upper control limit or below the lower control limit by chance is slightly more than 0.001, or one out of a thousand. Therefore, the probability of any point falling beyond either control limit by chance is 0.002, or approximately two out of a thousand. This is such a small probability that we look for a special or assignable cause when points fall beyond the control limits.

Occasionally, there are high-risk situations that may involve a closer review of the data. One way to ensure that review is to move the control limits into two standard deviations (2-sigma). For example, hospital laboratory departments that have used control charts in the past have traditionally used 2-sigma limits. When the sigma limit is reduced from three to two, the probability of a point falling beyond either control limit by chance is increased to approximately 0.05, or 5 out of a hundred (0.025 probability above and 0.025 below). In some cases even though a 2-sigma level is chosen, this probability may be increased even further with certain types of data. Because of this, there are many experts that recommend three standard deviations even for high-risk situations. For additional information on this topic, refer to Balestracci's (1998) publication.

Step 6: Review the Control Chart and Revise the Control Limits if Necessary

Once the initial calculations have been performed, the data may be displayed on the control chart. At this point, the steps outlined in chapter 3 regarding the interpretation of control charts should be reviewed to determine if the process is in control. As a reminder, if a sample falls outside of the control limits there is reason to believe that a special cause is present. Further, we expect the samples to exhibit a random ordering within these limits. If a group of samples shows a pattern, we also have reason to believe that a special cause is present.

To review the theory behind control charts and their control limits, refer to Figure 7.2, which shows a normal curve. This normal curve may represent bell-shaped data gathered to illustrate the performance of a process. In considering common and special cause variation, we are interested in knowing if special causes are influencing the process. If so, this is an indication that the process has changed in some way.

The normal distribution is identified by two factors—the *mean*, which is a measure of location, and the *standard deviation* or *range*, which shows the width of the data set. In this case, the standard deviation (sigma) is noted at the 3-sigma level. What we really want to know is, has the location and/or the width changed? If so, our process has

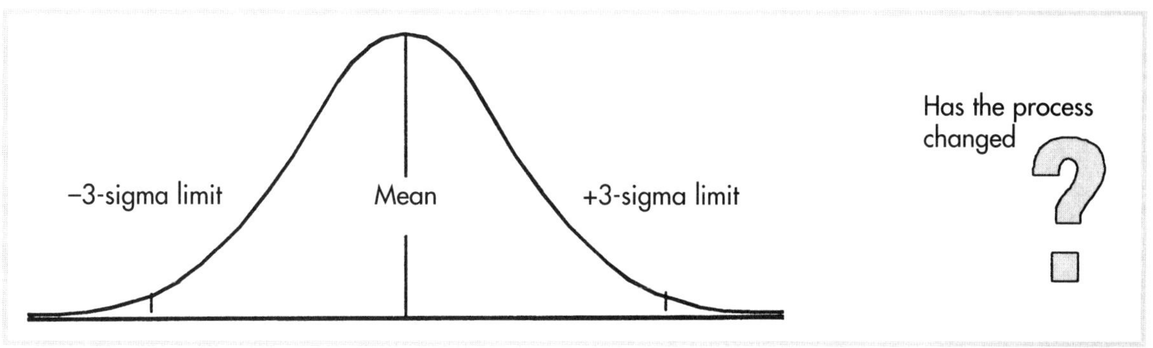

Used with permission from Gregory Gruska.

Figure 7.2. The normal curve.

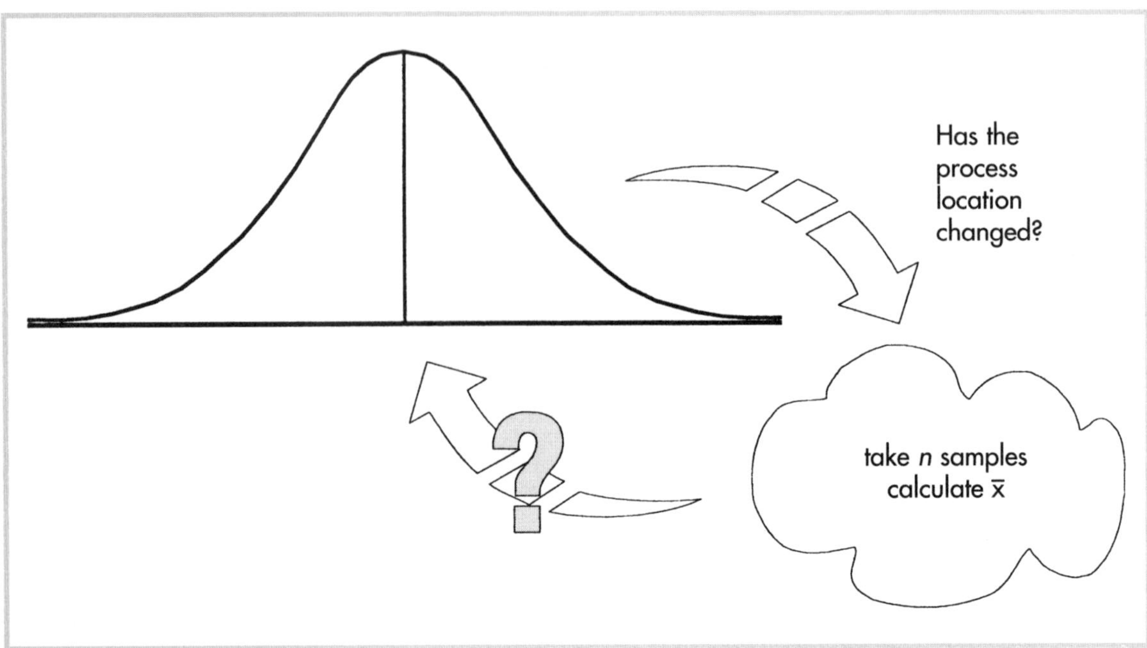
Has the
process
location
changed?
take n samples
calculate $\bar{x}$

Used with permission from Gregory Gruska.

Figure 7.3. Taking a sample from the population.

probably changed. It is usually not feasible to measure the entire process again and again to see if the width or location has changed, so instead, we take a sample and calculate a mean. Figure 7.3 shows the process of taking a sample from the population to see if the location has changed.

How likely is it that the mean of the sample will match the population mean if the process hasn't changed? The answer is that it is unlikely. Think about the crime rate for a certain community. If nothing has been done to reduce crime the process of criminal activity is likely to stay the same. However, the crime figures that are gathered each month will rarely be exactly the same. We expect that they will fluctuate even if the system has not changed. This is common cause variability.

Shewhart began with the assumption that the process is "in-statistical-control" or has not changed. When reviewing control charts we start off with the assumption that the process is in-statistical-control (that is, innocent till proven guilty) until we see special cause variation, which may mean that the process has changed.

If an out-of-control situation is noted, it should be investigated to determine if there is an assignable cause for the process variation. If it is determined that action may be taken to eliminate the special cause variability in the future, the control limits may be recalculated from the remaining samples. If an assignable cause cannot be identified as an out-of-control situation, or if there is no action taken to correct the situation, the control limits should not be recalculated.

Step 7: Implement and Monitor the Control Chart

The control chart is now ready to be used on an ongoing basis. It should be reviewed regularly for out-of-control (unstable) situations. Remember that out-of-control situations may not necessarily be negative. It is possible for a special cause to result in a positive outcome, such as a decrease in patient wait-times. In addition, it is possible for a process to be in statistical control—or stable—(exhibiting only common cause variation) and still not be acceptable. In those cases, the underlying system must be examined and changed. For example, if the average patient wait-time in the outpatient center is 20 minutes with an upper control limit of 45 minutes, it is possible those times are not acceptable to the patients. If a new service-provider agreement is signed that guarantees that patients will be seen in 20 minutes or less, our control chart shows us that this is impossible without changing the system. Assuming that we decide to take action, as mentioned in Step 6, if the process changes, the control limits should be recalculated.

When addressing a process to be changed, the tools and techniques presented in chapter 8 may be used. For example, a process that is experiencing a trend of increased errors may be addressed by flowcharting the process to determine the existing procedures. This may be followed by a root cause analysis to determine the reasons behind the increased errors, and benchmarking the same process at other *best-practice* organizations. Finally, a new flowchart outlining the way the process should be performed may be created. Once the new procedures have been implemented—either on a trial basis or full-scale basis—the control chart should be monitored to determine if the changes resulted in an improvement. Ultimately, as mentioned earlier, if the changes result in new control limits, the control chart should be revised to reflect the new limits.

EXERCISE

1. Brainstorm a list of four possible variables to be measured. Use the following grid to help identify one variable to measure. Assign point values based on the given scale. This scale may be modified for your own circumstances in future use.

Point Scale

0—No

1—Somewhat

2—Yes

	Variable #1:	Variable #2:	Variable #3:	Variable #4:
Is variable part of a key organizational process?				
Is variable part of a high-risk procedure?				
Is variable part of a high-volume procedure?				
Is variable part of a problem-prone area?				
Are data inexpensive to gather?				
Are data non-time consuming to gather?				
Is there a good potential for improvement?				
Total:				

2. Now that you've identified the variable to be measured, determine the sample size and frequency. The first step in this decision is the determination of the type of data you will be gathering—attribute or variable.

   The variable to be measured is: ______________________

   Data type: Attribute Variable

   Sample size: _________________

   Sample frequency: ________________

3. Review the flowchart in chapter 4 to determine the appropriate control chart.

   Control chart: ______________________

Reference

Balestracci, D. 1998. "Data 'Sanity': Statistical Thinking Applied to Everyday Data." *Special Publication.* ASQ Statistics Division.

CHAPTER 8

Integration of Control Charts with Other Quality Tools

Many of the quality tools are meant to work together. This chapter provides a brief presentation of some commonly used quality tools, and then presents the integration between the various tools, with particular emphasis on the use of control charts.

Check Sheet

The check sheet is one of the most basic quality tools. It was used long before quality improvement became popular. In fact, if your organization is not using any of the quality tools, chances are you have been using a check sheet and perhaps even calling it by a different name. The check sheet is used to gather data. It is simply a grid made up of rows and columns. Generally, the columns are labeled with various category names, while the rows may be labeled according to another designation such as the shift, date, or person gathering the data. The data are then recorded on the check sheet by placing a tick mark or a numeric value in the category column each time something that corresponds with the category has occurred. Figure 8.1 shows an example of a completed check sheet. This check sheet was used to determine why patients

<table>
<tr><th></th><th>Discharge instructions were not adequately explained to patient.</th><th>Patient did not get prescription filled.</th><th>Patient did not make a follow-up appointment with physician.</th><th>Other</th></tr>
<tr><td>Week 1</td><td>|</td><td>|||</td><td></td><td>|</td></tr>
<tr><td>Week 2</td><td></td><td>||</td><td>|</td><td>|</td></tr>
<tr><td>Week 3</td><td>|</td><td>||||/</td><td></td><td></td></tr>
<tr><td>Week 4</td><td>||</td><td>||</td><td></td><td>|</td></tr>
</table>

Figure 8.1. Check sheet to be used to find out why patient returned to emergency Department within 72 hours of first visit.

returned to the Emergency Department for treatment within 72 hours of their first visit. In this case, the reception clerk asked the patient questions relating to each of the four categories listed. Every affirmative answer received a tick mark in the corresponding column.

Check sheets help bring reliability—or consistency—to the data gathering process because if an individual has been given a clear understanding of the categories, the task of gathering data according to the categories becomes very consistent among data gatherers. The check sheet also saves time and money over many other data gathering methods because it is very easy to place a check mark in a column rather than listing items each time they occur.

Operational Definition

Even though many organizations use check sheets, they frequently forget one of the most important things about the check sheet. The check sheet should be accompanied with training for the people who will be using it to gather the data and should include an *operational definition*. The operational definition is a quality tool that helps reduce bias and errors in the data gathering process. The operational definition is simply a sentence that communicates important information to the data gatherer so that data are gathered the same way every time, even if there is more than one person gathering data. There are generally four elements to an operational definition. Fortunately, they are easy to remember because they form the acronym ABCD.

Audience: Who is being measured?

Behavior: What is being measured?

Condition: How is the measurement taking place?

Definition: Are there any terms that should be further defined?

The first three categories (A–C) relate to the data gathering process. The last category (Definition) relates to the A–C above it. It is meant to remind you to clarify any items that may cause confusion and need to be further defined. One of the things we can do with D is to remember to read A–C to others and see if they all have the same understanding of the data gathering process. Another thing we can do with D is to ask questions such as, Does C give us the A and B that we expect? In other words, does the condition under which the data are being gathered allow us to obtain the behavior information we anticipate from the people we want to obtain information from? This step may seem like a waste of time but it really isn't. People frequently think they are gathering certain types of information, when in fact, they are not gathering the data they intended. The example of the need for an operational definition was first presented in chapter 7. In that instance, it was found that various people were measuring surgical start-time in different ways. In that case, an operational definition that may assist them could be the following:

Audience: The patients undergoing surgery from January 7–14 at XYZ Hospital

Behavior: The actual start-time of the surgery

Condition: The RN will record the time the surgery started on the check sheet

Definition: Surgical start-time is defined as the time the first incision is made

Think for a moment about how you might write an operational definition for the reception clerk completing the check sheet in the Emergency Room example previously described. Write your operational definition:

Audience:

Behavior:

Condition:

Definition:

If all individuals involved in the data gathering process either assist in developing the operational definition or are informed of the operational definition prior to gathering data, the data are more likely to be gathered in a uniform manner that will reduce possible bias in the measurement. Unfortunately, even the best techniques will not guarantee that there is not some bias in the data. According to Deming as quoted by Neave, "There is no true value of anything" (Neave 1990, 113). The goal therefore is to reduce the amount of bias—and an operational definition will assist toward that end.

Check Sheet and Operational Definition Use with Control Charts

The data that are placed on a control chart come from various sources. Sometimes information may be manually obtained from files, gathered by observation, or extracted from computer databases. In many cases, no matter what kinds of data are being gathered, a check sheet can often be adapted to fit the circumstances. When a check sheet is accompanied with an operational definition, it increases the probability that the data gathered for the control chart are reliable and valid. Remember that the control chart is only as good as the data that are used to develop it. If the data are flawed, the control chart is useless.

Process Flowchart

Most healthcare organizations are familiar with process flowcharting and have used it for some time. The flowchart visually shows the steps involved in a process. There are four commonly used symbols in flowcharts, the oval (beginning/end of process), the rectangle (activity), the diamond (decision), and the circle (connects with other processes). The arrows that connect these shapes indicate the flow of the process.

One of the things that is often missing from a flowchart—and the process itself—is the incorporation of measurement of the process. Key organizational processes should have designated places for measurement within the flowchart. Measurement may be indicated by rectangles (the activity of taking the measurement) and diamonds (reviewing and acting upon the measurement) that are placed throughout the process. The importance of the diamond immediately (or shortly) following the measurement activity indicates that the measurement is evaluated as a part of the process rather than at a later date. Think of this as "taking the pulse of the process." There are two primary options for measurement within a process flowchart.

Upstream: Measurement points throughout the process

Downstream: Measurement at the end of the process

Upstream Measurement

Upstream measurement is indicated by measurement points throughout the process. The key to upstream measurement is to evaluate the data immediately. If there are problems in the process they can be pinpointed and addressed quickly. Most organizations do downstream (or outcome) measures. However, if problems frequently appear in the downstream (outcome) measurement, measurement activities may be placed at key intervals upstream to see where the problem starts to occur. Think about a polluted river in which a downstream measurement detects a contaminant. If measurement points are placed in several upstream locations, the place at which the pollution enters the river may be pinpointed.

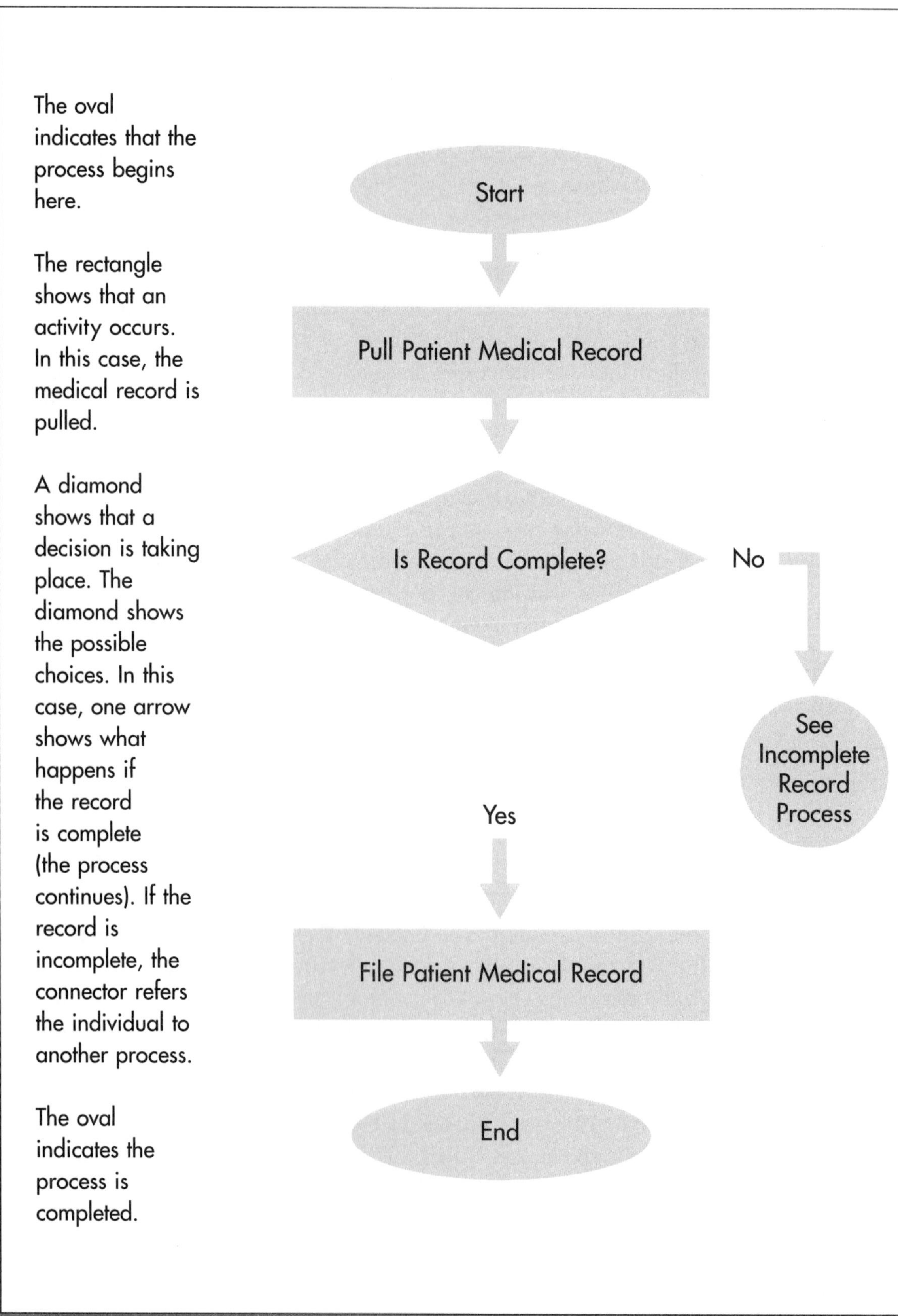
The oval indicates that the process begins here.
The rectangle shows that an activity occurs. In this case, the medical record is pulled.
A diamond shows that a decision is taking place. The diamond shows the possible choices. In this case, one arrow shows what happens if the record is complete (the process continues). If the record is incomplete, the connector refers the individual to another process.
The oval indicates the process is completed.
Start
Pull Patient Medical Record
Is Record Complete?
No
See Incomplete Record Process
Yes
File Patient Medical Record
End

DOWNSTREAM MEASUREMENT

Downstream measurement is the measurement that takes place at the end of a process. Organizations have traditionally measured exclusively downstream, ignoring upstream measurement. Downstream measurement is important and should not be abandoned, because it is the ultimate measure that customers often have access to. However, if it is the only measurement taking place, organizations miss opportunities for improvement within the process. For example, some healthcare organizations measure cesarian rates (downstream) without really looking at the upstream measurements that may affect the process. If the organization's cesarian rates increased for no apparent reason, upstream measurement may be used to look at the risk factors of the patients entering the system. One organization did this and found that in the preceding year several smaller hospitals had begun sending higher-risk patients to the larger hospital, thus increasing the larger hospital's cesarian rate. Without upstream measurement, organizations frequently resort to the *easy solution*, which is usually to blame the people within the system—in this case the physicians had been blamed.

Figure 8.2 shows an upstream measurement of patient satisfaction within the process of treating the inpatient. In this example, it was decided that rather than wait for the patient survey to be

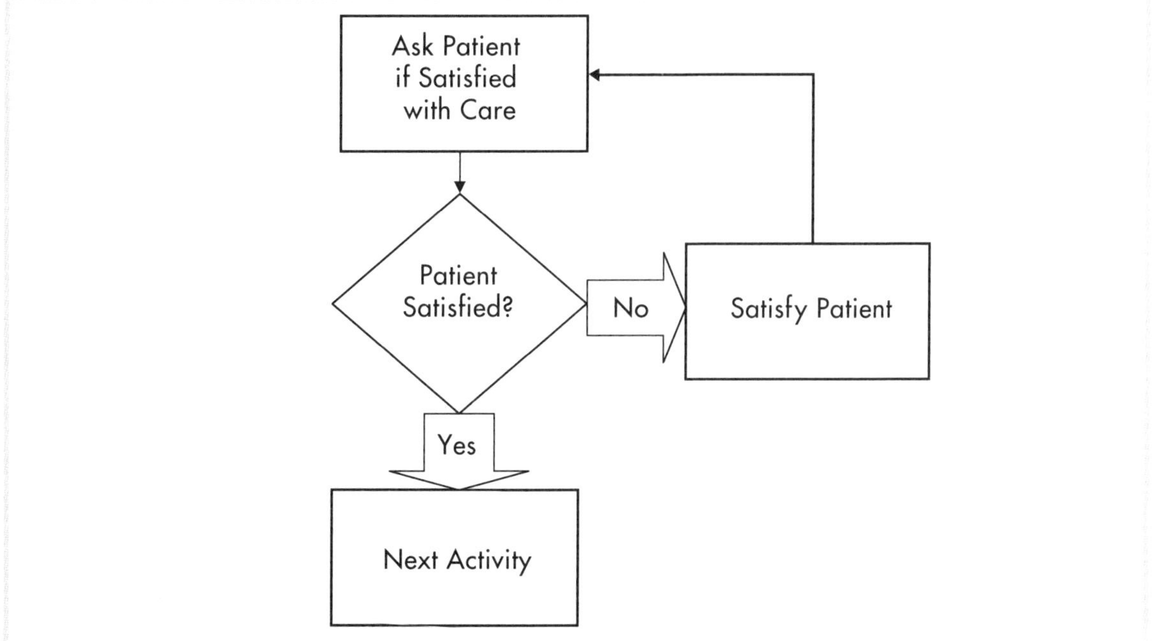

Figure 8.2. Flowchart with upstream measurement.

returned by mail (by which time the opportunity for improvement would have long since passed), an upstream measurement was inserted within the process to be performed by a trained volunteer. This particular hospital already had volunteers who visited the floor with a hospitality cart. The volunteers were given a grid with each room number and the possibility to place a check in one of several boxes. The boxes related to areas of satisfaction that included various factors that appeared to be problems according to the past satisfaction surveys. Upon entering each room, the volunteer asked each patient several questions relating to the areas identified on the grid. If a patient was dissatisfied, it was simply a matter of the volunteer checking the appropriate box. Later in the day, the forms were given to a hospital employee who visited the patients who were dissatisfied to see if there was anything that could be done. Finally, after the patient left the hospital, a survey was sent to the home to capture downstream data.

Process Flowcharting and Control Charts

One of the best ways to display and evaluate the measurement data taken within a process is to use a control chart. In the situation of patient satisfaction just mentioned, the number of items indicating dissatisfaction on the check sheets may be displayed on an attribute control chart. The organization is now in an excellent position to see if its new upstream measurement is effective, and can continue to monitor patient satisfaction levels—both upstream and downstream—over time.

Cause-and-Effect Diagram

The cause-and-effect diagram is known by several different names. It is called the *Ishikawa Diagram* after the man who invented it, the *fishbone* diagram after its appearance, and the cause-and-effect diagram after its use. It is most closely identified with a root cause analysis. Hospitals that have reported a *sentinel event* are required by the Joint Commission to do a root cause analysis. A sentinel event as defined by the Joint Commission as ". . . an unexpected occurrence involving death or serious physical or psychological injury, or the risk thereof" (Joint Commission Perspectives, 1998, 2). It is therefore important that individuals in hospital settings be familiar with this quality tool. The time to learn to use an Ishikawa Diagram is not immediately following a sentinel event. This is one tool that may be used frequently in an organization's ongoing problem solving activities; therefore, when a sentinel event does occur, the individuals in the hospital will be experienced in its use.

A sample outline of a fishbone diagram is shown in Figure 8.3.

Notice there is one large "backbone" along the middle of the chart. This indicates the effect or the problem. A statement of the problem is generally placed at the end of this arrow where the word "effect" appears. The five "large bones" indicate five possible categories of causes. These five causes are to be used as a starting point for an Ishikawa Diagram. Initially, all five categories should be considered as possible causes. If any are not appropriate for the situation, they may be discarded. Conversely, if there are other large causes that were not included, they can be included as *large bones.* Once this has been accomplished, the next step is to brainstorm the contributing factors to the problem along each large bone. As factors are stated they should be added as *small bones* along the appropriate large bone. Each time a factor is added, a series of *why questions* are posed to the group. As these *whys* are answered, the answer is placed as a bone that is an offshoot of the bone that spawned it.

For example, an organization's Emergency Department (ED) may want to probe the root causes of patients returning for treatment within three days for the same diagnosis.

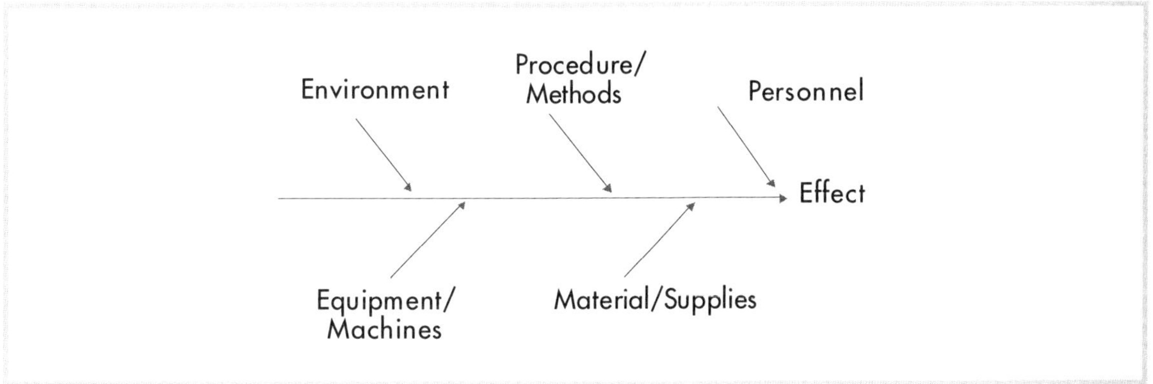

Figure 8.3. Ishikawa Diagram.

Steps:

1. Draw the backbone on flipchart paper and write a problem statement at the end of the bone as shown in Figure 8.4.
2. Review the five commonly used *large bones* and determine which are appropriate for your situation. Place those bones on the flipchart paper.
3. Decide if there are any *large bones* that should be added. If so, place them on the diagram. In the case of our Emergency Department example, we decided to use the bones shown in Figure 8.5.
4. Start with one large bone and ask, Why is the *fill in name of large bone* a cause of the problem? Write down the first thing mentioned. Hint: If you place the response on sticky notes, you can easily move them around if you decide they fit better in other places. Using our ED example, let's begin with the large bone of *patient.*
   a. Why is the patient a cause of a return to the ED? Perhaps the patient did not follow treatment instructions.
5. Continue to ask why until there is a natural end.

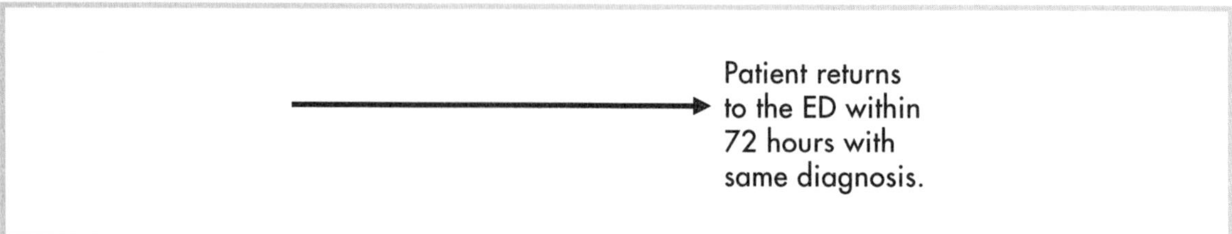

Figure 8.4. Beginning an Ishikawa Diagram.

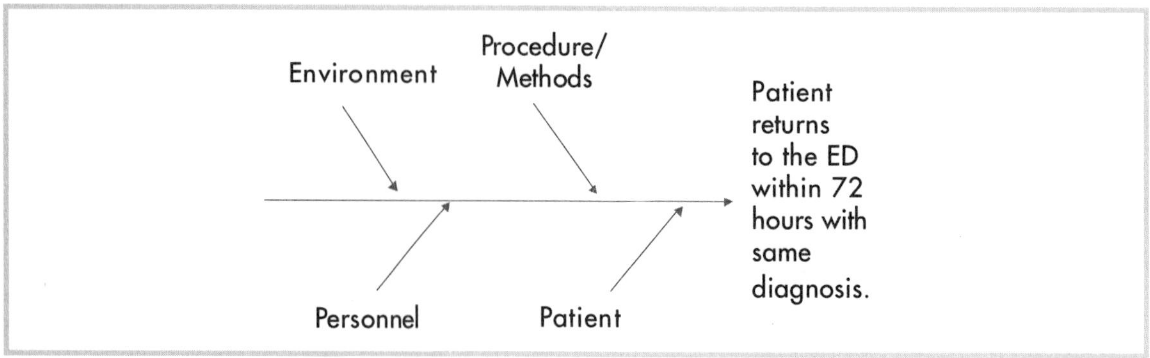

Figure 8.5. Large bones on an Ishikawa Diagram.

a. Why did the patient not follow treatment instructions?
   Perhaps the patient did not understand the instructions.
b. Why did patient not understand instructions?
   Perhaps the instructions were not explained well or not explained at all.
c. Why were the instructions not explained well or not explained at all?
   No one is assigned the responsibility of explaining the treatment instructions to the patient. At present time, everyone knows it should be done, but no one has the direct responsibility of doing so.

At this point the whys just naturally end. It is often said that the "why question" must be asked approximately five times before a root cause emerges.

Figure 8.6 illustrates the portion of the Ishikawa Diagram that was discussed. This process will continue on each of the bones until several root causes are determined.

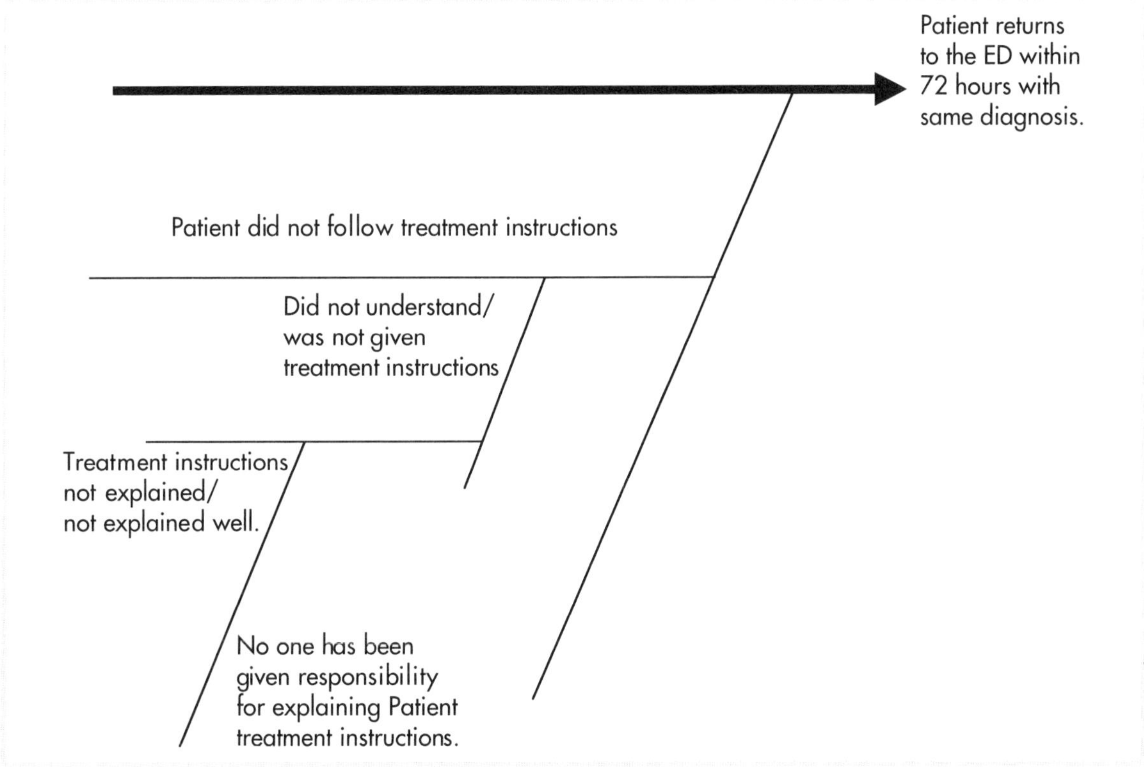

Figure 8.6. Section of an Ishikawa Diagram.

This tool has been used by many organizations for numerous situations. It has proven to be a very effective method for determining root causes. There are also precautions to be taken when using this tool.

1. Don't let your root cause end by blaming a person. In the preceding situation, it would have been easy to stop the analysis by blaming the patient for not following instructions, or an employee for not administering treatment instructions, and ending at that step. However, the Ishikawa Diagram should never end with blame of a person. In situations such as this, the next question that is asked is what in the system allowed the person to take the actions that were made? Another way to ask this is, why did this occur? Obviously, in this case, there was a lack of responsibility for giving the instructions. Often a primary reason for a breakdown in a process involving an individual is a lack of training.
2. Don't go into a root cause analysis with the problem already mentally solved. Predetermined solutions will make the root cause ineffective. It is important that the group feels free to explore any possible cause that arises. Sometimes group members have to make an effort to prevent bias from entering into the analysis. For example, if the people doing the root cause in the previous situation already decided that the real root cause is lack of training, and the solution is to train everyone, that bias will run throughout the discussion, prohibiting the group from exploring any other options. Sometimes a group can handle this by identifying possible biases before proceeding and making an effort to look further than the identified solutions.
3. Occasionally groups will stop short of the root cause by not asking *why* enough times. These Ishikawa Diagrams appear to be just skimming the surface on the root cause. As mentioned earlier, it is often the case that the why question should be asked at least five times.
4. In order to determine the root cause, it is sometimes necessary to explore "sacred cows." People should feel free to explore any possible root cause without feeling that some areas are off-limits. Sometimes people become very defensive when others verbally tread on their territory. It is very important to put defensiveness aside, as this will prohibit a good analysis. Conversely, it is extremely important to depersonalize all areas—especially sensitive

ones—and concentrate on the system without placing individual blame. Sometimes an outside moderator will help in these situations. Talk ahead of time about the possible barriers to open and honest discussion. Agree to set aside defensiveness, avoid finger-pointing and discuss any other necessary ground rules. If sensitive items are being discussed, a confidentiality agreement should be reached among members of the group.

5. If you are using the Ishikawa Diagram for a sentinel event, make sure that leadership is part of the root cause discussion. Not only does the Joint Commission recommend leadership involvement, a more practical reason is that leadership may not be open to any recommendations made by the team unless they were involved in the analysis. However, it is usually not a good idea for top leadership to lead or dominate the discussion because of the bias that may result. For example, one hospital went through the root cause analysis without leadership involvement and came up with solutions that were then rejected by top management. The organization decided to do the root cause analysis again with leadership involvement, but this time the CEO led the root cause analysis. Is it any surprise that the solutions were the ones the leadership had in mind in the first place? The root cause that emerged from the second analysis ended up blaming the individuals in one particular department. Obviously, both situations were handled incorrectly. Often the best mixture includes the people who have the closest involvement in the process, as well as one or two members of the leadership team.

6. Remember that the Ishikawa Diagram is a qualitative tool—we are gathering words. One of the criticisms about qualitative information is its subjectivity. It is therefore extremely important that the root causes identified by the Ishikawa diagram be verified through actual data analysis. That leads us naturally to the Pareto chart and, ultimately, to the control charts.

Pareto Chart

The Pareto chart may be used by itself or in conjunction with several other quality tools. Its purpose is to display data in a manner that separates the major contributors to problems from the minor contributors to problems. The whole idea is that as long as we are making the effort to address a problem, we should tackle the areas that will give us the biggest payback. For example, when using the Ishikawa Diagram in the Emergency Department example, we may determine that there are five root causes. Even though we have identified these possible root causes, we do not have objective data to verify if they are really root causes. In addition, we don't know the impact of each of the causes. For example, one cause may contribute approximately 70 percent of the problem, whereas another may contribute only 3 percent. It would not make sense to address both causes with the same vigor. Therefore, we move directly from the Ishikawa Diagram to the use of a Pareto chart to supply us with the information necessary to make data-driven decisions.

The Pareto chart is based on the Pareto principle that states that 80 percent of the problem comes from 20 percent of the causes. In actual practice, these percentages don't usually hold true—however, the general principle is the same. Not every cause contributes equally to every problem. It is important to determine those causes that will have the biggest effect upon the problem if addressed properly.

The activities of creating a Pareto chart are divided into two major categories: before data gathering and after data gathering. The steps in both activities follow.

Before Data Gathering:

1. Determine the data classifications.
2. Decide how importance is to be determined (i.e., frequency, time, cost).
3. Train/orient the data collectors.
4. Begin to gather data (use check sheet and operational definition if applicable).

After Data Gathering:

5. Review data for potential problems.
6. Total and rank the categories in descending order.
7. Compute relative and cumulative frequencies of categories.
8. Display the data on a bar graph.
9. Identify the most important causes of the problem.

A detailed discussion of each of the steps follows.

Before Data Gathering:

1. Determine the data classifications.

   Data classifications are the categories that will be used to gather data. When a Pareto chart follows an Ishikawa Diagram, the categories are derived from the root causes identified in the Ishikawa analysis. Other possible ways to determine categories are through brainstorming, past databased history, and personal knowledge.

2. Decide how importance is to be determined (i.e., frequency, time, cost).

   Once the data classifications have been identified, the next step is to decide how the importance of the categories will be determined. In most cases the importance is determined by frequency—or how often the situations identified in each of the categories occur. In the Emergency Department example previously discussed, it would be important to determine the frequency in which patients did not get their prescriptions filled or did not follow treatment instructions. Sometimes, however, importance may be determined by means other than frequency, such as time or cost. For example, if we were exploring the reasons for delays in the outpatient center, one category may be that the computer system is not operational. If the center was extremely dependent upon the computer system, even an occasional failure of the system may cause tremendous problems. In this case, it might be relevant to determine importance based on time—how much of a time delay occurs each time the computer system goes down—rather than frequency (how often it goes down).

3. Train/orient the data collectors.

   Data collection should not begin without an orientation of people who will be collecting the data. Ideally, these people should be involved in the discussion at an early stage—even helping to develop the check sheet and the operational definition. This step is very important in assuring reliability and validity of the data collected.

4. Begin to gather data (use check sheet and operational definition if applicable).

   As mentioned earlier, a check sheet and operational definition will assist greatly in the data collection. If it is not appropriate to use a check sheet, an operational definition should still be used to guide the data gathering.

After Data Gathering:

5. Review data for potential problems.

   Review the data with a critical eye. It is often very difficult to catch a built-in bias in the data; however, think about what could have gone wrong during the data collection and test the data quality against a list of potential problems. Look for unusual values and verify that they did, indeed, occur. Once you're satisfied with the quality of the data, the analysis may begin.

6. Total and rank the categories in descending order.

   Each category should be totaled. If (in Step 2) the importance was determined by frequency, each category's total frequency should be obtained, and placed in order from most frequent to least frequent. If importance was determined by another method such as time or cost, these should also be totaled by category and placed in descending order. An example of this step, using the data gathered with the check sheet in the beginning of this chapter, is displayed in Figure 8.7.

	Patient did not get prescription filled.	Discharge instructions were not adequately explained to patient.	Other	Patient did not make a follow-up appointment with physician.
Week 1	|||	|	|	
Week 2	||		|	|
Week 3	~~||||~~	|		
Week 4	||	||	|	
Total	12	4	3	1

Figure 8.7. Check sheet for Emergency Department.

7. Compute relative and cumulative frequencies of categories.

   If you have a computer package that creates Pareto charts, the program will do the remaining steps. However, if you are creating a Pareto chart by hand, you will need to calculate the relative and cumulative frequencies for each category. The *relative frequency* is simply the frequency in each category divided by the total frequency. The *cumulative frequency* is obtained by adding each relative frequency to the previous cumulative frequency when placed in descending order. Figure 8.8 shows the relative and cumulative frequencies of each of the categories.

8. Display the data on a bar graph.

   The results of the calculations that were performed in Step 7 are now displayed in a bar graph and shown in Figure 8.9. The relative

	Patient did not get prescription filled.	Discharge instructions were not adequately explained to patient.	Other	Patient did not make a follow-up appointment with physician.
Week 1	|||	|	|	
Week 2	||		|	|
Week 3	~~||||~~	|		
Week 4	||	||	|	
Total	12	4	3	1
Relative Frequency	12/20 = 0.60	4/20 = 0.20	3/20 = 0.15	1/20 = 0.05
Cumulative Frequency	0.60	0.60 + 0.20 = 0.80	0.80 + 0.15 = 0.95	0.95 + 0.05 = 1.00

Figure 8.8. Pareto chart calculations on check sheet.

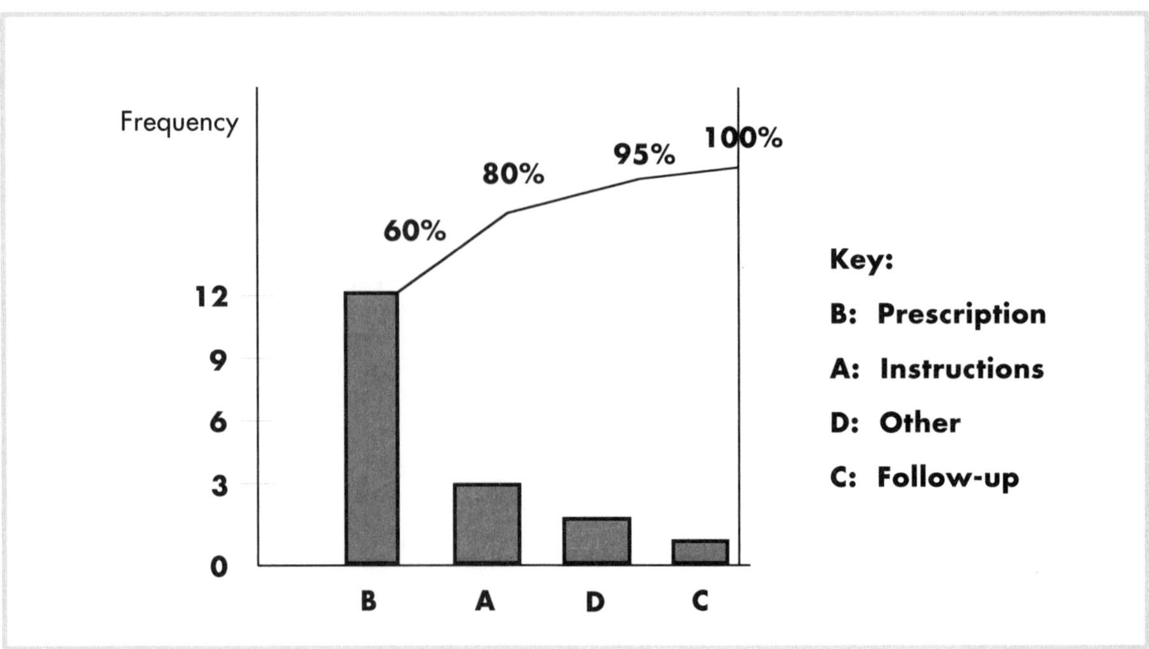

Figure 8.9. Pareto chart for Emergency Department.

frequencies are shown on the vertical axis, while the horizontal axis designates the various categories. The columns are shown in descending order. The cumulative frequencies are shown in an arc over the top of the bars, indicating how much of the problem will be solved as each bar is addressed. Therefore, if the problem of getting a prescription filled is adequately addressed, 60 percent of the total problem of return visits to the ED will be addressed. If we can address both the prescription problem and the treatment instructions, 80 percent of the problem will be addressed, and so on.

9. Identify the most important causes of the problem.

   Unless there is an unusual, compelling reason to do otherwise, the important causes are identified as the first bar, and all subsequent bars, in descending order. Therefore, in the example given, the team should now address the first cause (prescription not filled) and move along to the other causes as needed.

Control Chart Use with Pareto Charts

After items have been identified for improvement, it is important to place a tool in the system to see if the changes are effective. This is an ideal use for a control chart. The control chart should be developed using data before any changes have taken place. Once changes are made, data should continue to be gathered, and the control chart should be monitored to see if the changes are effective. Obviously, if the changes are not working, other ways to solve the problem should be pursued.

Fitting the Tools Together

This summary shows the way the tools discussed in this chapter will fit together when addressing everyday problems or even a sentinel event. When doing a root cause analysis to be shown to the Joint Commission after a sentinel event, the following tool structure may be used; however, JCAHO also requires that a literature review be performed in addition to using the tools outlined in this chapter. We have indicated the literature review step in the benchmarking designation. *Benchmarking* is the process of looking for a better way to do a process by comparing the way we do the process to other organizations—preferably those that have a reputation for being the best-in-class at what they do.

Quality Improvement Steps/Root Cause Analysis

1	Flowchart the process as it is being done now.	Process flowchart
2	Do a cause-and-effect diagram with involvement of both leadership and the people involved in the process.	Ishikawa Diagram
3	Follow the "before data gathering" Pareto chart steps.	Pareto chart
4	Place the Pareto chart categories on a check sheet for data gathering.	Check sheet
5	Create an operational definition to accompany the check sheet.	Operational definition
6	While the data gathering is taking place, search the literature and comparative databases to see how others	

continued

continued

	are performing the process and how it compares to your performance.	Benchmarking/Literature review
7	Gather data, then complete the "after data gathering" Pareto chart steps.	Pareto chart
8	Based on the results of the Pareto chart, determine possible solutions. Pilot test a solution and examine the process performance by using a control chart.	Control chart
9	If the control chart shows that the change worked, standardize the change by creating a new process flowchart. Include continued measurement and improvement within the process.	Process flowchart and control chart

EXERCISE 8.1

Complete the following grid by placing the appropriate tool in the box on the right. You may use some tools more than once.

What You Want to Do:	Tool You Will Use:
Find out to what degree things are causing a particular problem.	
Gather data in an efficient manner.	
Determine possible root causes of a problem.	
Understand the steps involved in a process.	
Learn what others are doing in the field regarding a specified process.	
Standardize a change in the process.	
Monitor data over time.	
Help ensure the data are gathered by everyone in the same manner.	
Help lead a group discussion to determine inputs into a problem.	
Display the inputs in problems in a manner that makes it clear which ones are the biggest causes of the problem.	
See if the change you made to the process has improved the process.	

EXERCISE 8.2

1. Think of a process you perform in your organization. Flowchart its macro (major) steps.
2. Think about where an upstream and downstream measurement might occur. Place both measurements into a new process flowchart.
3. Determine how you will gather data for both measurements. Choose the appropriate control chart for one of the measurements of your choice.

   Upstream: The thing to be measured is: ____________________

   The appropriate control chart is: ____________________

   Downstream: The thing to be measured is: ____________________

   The appropriate control chart is: ____________________
4. Write an operational definition for one of the measurements.

   Audience: ______________________________

   Behavior: ______________________________

   Condition: ______________________________

   Definition: ______________________________

References

Ishikawa, K. 1985. *What is Total Quality Control? The Japanese Way*. Englewood Cliffs, NJ: Prentice-Hall.

JCAHO. 1998. *Joint Commission Perspectives*. Oakbrook Terrace, IL: Joint Commission on Accreditation of Healthcare Organizations.

Neave, H. R. 1990. *The Deming Dimension*. Knoxville, TN: SPC Press, Inc.

CHAPTER 9

Using Quality Tools to Meet JCAHO's Performance Improvement Standards

References to the Joint Commission have been integrated throughout this book. This chapter, however, is dedicated to providing an overview of JCAHO's PI Standards, and linking the tools discussed previously with the specific standards. As individuals in healthcare organizations are well aware, the standards are updated regularly—often annually; therefore, a direct reference/footnote for each standard mentioned throughout the book is not practical and has not been provided.

As mentioned previously, JCAHO's references to quality have evolved over the years. A number of years ago, *quality assurance* was the terminology used (an overview of QA is provided in chapter 1). This was a "first step" toward quality. Unfortunately, many of the efforts in this area were not grounded in theory. In addition, most hospital personnel were not trained to take on the new roles and philosophies of quality. Finally, it was decided that the terminology itself was not appropriate. We don't want to give the impression that we can *assure* quality—especially when facing malpractice litigation. Quality assurance is also counter to a continuous improvement philosophy because the terminology implies that once quality is assured, we're done with improvement—we need only maintain the course. In fairness to the healthcare industry, this was new ground that was being covered.

Quality assurance then evolved into quality assessment. This was quite handy because the initials didn't change—therefore, all of the manuals and plans that healthcare organizations are required to keep did not have to be revised! Unfortunately, as its name implies, the assessment aspect of quality stopped short of continuously improving quality. The terminology suggested that the emphasis was on measurement (assessment), which created a plethora of data, but very little in the way of proactive improvement activities.

Performance improvement appears to be here to stay for a while. Healthcare organizations are beginning to embrace the idea of improvement for improvement's sake. They also see an opportunity to reduce the sheer volume of data collection, and are realizing that they can gather data they can really use. The PI standards give much of the decision-making power back to healthcare organizations by letting them decide exactly how they will fulfill the PI standards. The increased Joint Commission emphasis, however, is on data-driven decision making, use of statistical tools, and interdisciplinary activities. This emphasis is grounded in theory and is very similar to Deming's philosophies.

JCAHO Performance Improvement Themes

The overall themes in the PI standards are as follows:

1. Leadership is highly involved in PI activities.
2. The approach to performance improvement is planned, collaborative, interdisciplinary, systematic, and organization-wide.
3. The data being gathered are prioritized and systematically obtained.
4. The data from the measurements are collected over time and compared with current data from other sources.
5. Statistical methods are utilized. Common and special cause variation are examined, and action is taken when appropriate.
6. A format is followed for the redesign of existing processes and the design of new processes. The format includes baseline performance expectations.

A detailed discussion of each area follows.

Leadership Involvement

1. Leadership is highly involved in PI activities.

   As mentioned in chapter 2, as of 1999, leadership is held responsible for implementation of the PI standards. Therefore, many of the deficiencies in the PI standards will be scored against the leadership standards. This represents a major change from previous years. The first responsibility for PI is for leadership to design a process to perform performance improvement. The process should be outlined in the PI Plan. Chapter 2 contains a PI Plan guideline based on JCAHO criteria. There should be a strong interrelationship between the PI Plan and the other plans required by JCAHO, such as the strategic plan, the information management plan, and the plan for the provision of patient care services.

   Leadership is also responsible for assuring that the structures are in place for PI to be effective. Leaders should evaluate existing improvement processes and make sure they provide a unified, organization-wide approach to quality. This includes assessing employee training needs regarding PI tools and techniques, and allocating adequate resources to conduct PI activities. Another important leadership responsibility is in determining the criteria for selection of improvement activities. One tool that may be used by leaders is a selection grid. A basic selection grid was described in chapter 7. Leadership may use a selection grid to prioritize improvement activities. The criteria for the grid are obtained by reviewing the strategic plan, regulatory requirements, and contractual obligations. These criteria are placed on the grid with a corresponding scoring range. Improvement options are then scored against the grid with the highest-scoring items becoming top priority for upcoming improvement efforts. A sample leadership selection grid is provided in Table 9.1.

   Another area of involvement for leadership is in a possible sentinel event. As mentioned earlier, JCAHO defines a sentinel event as, "an unexpected occurrence involving death or serious physical or psychological injury, or the risk thereof." Any JCAHO-accredited healthcare organization must take specific actions in the case of a sentinel event. The leadership of the organization must spearhead these steps and present evidence of active leadership involvement in the root cause analysis in order for the JCAHO to deem the root cause activity credible.

Table 9.1. Leadership Selection Grid

	Option meets Strategic Plan Objective #1 (Score 0 –5)	Option meets JCAHO PI Standard #xxx (Score 0 –5)	. . . and so on	Total
Improvement Option 1	1	3		12
Improvement Option 2	0	5		14
. . . and so on				

The Approach to Performance Improvement

2. The approach to performance improvement is planned, collaborative, interdisciplinary, systematic, and organization-wide.

   In order to have planned PI activities, the structure must be contained in a written document. The document is called the *PI Plan*. The plan must be implemented organization-wide. For example, when a JCAHO surveyor asks a dietary employee how he or she does performance improvement, the employee should be able to discuss the same methodology as the nursing employee. An example of a methodology that has been incorporated in many PI Plans is Deming's Plan, Do, Study, Act (PDSA) cycle, as discussed in chapter 2.

   The PI Plan should also emphasize the collaborative, interdisciplinary nature of PI activities. There must be evidence in improvement activities, committee minutes, and committee/team structures of employee representation across the organization. This does not eliminate the need for department-specific activities. There is still a need for performance improvement efforts in departments for processes that do not impact other departments. However, processes that span several departments or disciplines must have interdisciplinary representation when performance improvement activities occur.

   A helpful guide when thinking about systematic, interdisciplinary and collaborative activities is *The Democratic Corporation* by Russell Ackoff (1994). In this book, Ackoff discusses the systems approach to quality. The idea behind the systems approach is that choosing pieces of a process to improve will not necessarily result in a better process. In his famous "car" example, Ackoff discusses improving every piece of a car by benchmarking the best-in-class for each part. For example, the best engine, the best transmission, the best cooling system, and so on, are all purchased to assemble into the "best" car. Unfortunately, the pieces don't fit together—so instead of having the best car, we end up with a car that doesn't run! When improving the organization, it is not enough for each department to improve its own little world—because improvements in one may result in a negative impact on others. The key is to take a collaborative, interdisciplinary look at the entire process to find ways to make the whole organization better.

Prioritized and Systematically Obtained Data

3. The data being gathered are prioritized and systematically obtained.

   One of the ways to examine an organization's data is to perform a data inventory. A data inventory is one of the first tasks that should be undertaken in PI. The data inventory allows the leadership to make comparisons between what is presently being gathered and what should be gathered. In general, organizations tend to gather too much data or the wrong type of data.

Creating a Data Inventory

Healthcare organizations are inundated by data gathering activities. Unfortunately, the massive amounts of data do not generally translate in data-driven decisions. The data are often gathered inconsistently, analyzed poorly, and presented to a committee—where they are promptly stowed away with the committee minutes until a regulatory agency pays a visit. One of the main reasons we don't do a good job in using the data we gather is because we obtain so much data that it is overwhelming to determine where to begin in actually using the information generated by the data.

Most people remember a few years back when JCAHO required every area within a hospital to identify two indicators on which to gather data. Organizations that were already measuring things added the two indicators per area to their existing measurements. Then when

JCAHO dropped its two-indicator requirement, many healthcare organizations were afraid to stop measuring, so the measurement carried on . . . and on . . . and on! Recently, during a training session, one poor hospital librarian asked if she still had to keep track of the number of overdue books per month and the number of periodicals checked out per month. Those were her two indicators, and she had been faithfully recording the numbers on a little form for many, many years. The other common problem is the duplication of measurement within healthcare organizations. Frequently, two departments are measuring the same thing. The interesting thing is that frequently, the numbers don't even match!

A data inventory is designed to reduce the amount of data being gathered so the focus can be on gathering timely, valid, and reliable data. When the data quality is good, and the amount of data is not overwhelming, organizations can begin to actually use the data being gathered.

The steps in conducting a data inventory follow.

---

1. Review regulatory requirements, contractual obligations, and the organization's strategic plan to determine measures of performance.
2. Distribute the data inventory form.
3. Filter all data.
4. Create a data depository.

---

1. Review regulatory requirements, contractual obligations, and the organization's strategic plan to determine measures of performance.

   This step of the data inventory determines exactly what data should be gathered. At this point, a list is made of those indicators that are necessary for the organization. Ultimately, the data that are being gathered will be compared to this list and superfluous data will be eliminated. Requirements may include JCAHO, Health Care Financing Authority (HCFA), OSHA, state and local guidelines, issues concerning corporate compliance, and contractual obligations including managed care contracts. The strategic plan is also reviewed to determine the organization's strategic objectives and the corresponding measurements. Items also to be considered are high-volume, high-risk, and problem-prone areas. While reviewing all of

DATA INVENTORY FORM

Please complete this page *for each type* of data being gathered (make copies as necessary).

Name of person completing this form: ______________________________

Department/Committee/Team ______________________________

1. Please describe the type of data currently being gathered.

2. Exactly how are the data being gathered?

3. What is the data source?

4. How often are the data being gathered?

5. Who gathers the data?

6. Why are the data being gathered?

7. How are the data being used?

8. What type of analysis is being performed with the data?

9. Do you think it is necessary to continue to gather these data?

   _____ Yes _____ No Why? ______________________________

   ____

   ____

Please attach a sample of the data.

Figure 9.1.

the various requirements, keep in mind that some measurements may meet more than one requirement. For example, one measurement may fulfill requirements from several regulatory agencies, contractual obligations, and strategic plan objectives.

2. Distribute the data inventory form.

   Contact every team, committee, department, and person responsible for gathering data. Ask them to complete the questions shown in Figure 9.1 with samples of the data being gathered attached to the form.

3. Filter all data.

   Compare the data being gathered with the list of required data. When it appears that unnecessary data are being gathered, discuss the situation with the individuals who gather the data before arbitrarily eliminating the data. Winnow out duplicate data-gathering instances. Give people permission to stop gathering unnecessary data!

4. Create a data depository.

   The data depository is the one place that all data will be sent to. The data depository is monitored by the organization's data broker. The *data broker* is an individual responsible for maintaining a catalog and reference area for all of the organization's data. This person can standardize data-gathering procedures, create electronic files, and continue to streamline the data process. The departments within the organization that are designated to gather data will forward the data to the data depository. In addition, when data are needed, they are easily located by contacting the data broker.

A selection grid may also be used to help prioritize the data to be gathered. The categories on the selection grid are often based on the organization's strategic objectives, regulatory requirements, and contractual obligations.

JCAHO Required Measurements

There are some areas that are required by JCAHO for data collection. As of 1999, the required measurements for JCAHO are as follows:

1. Anesthesia, operative, and invasive and noninvasive procedures that place the patients at risk, including pre- and postoperative major discrepancies and adverse anesthesia occurrences.

2. Medication use, including significant medication errors and adverse drug reactions.
3. Use of blood and blood components and all confirmed transfusion reactions.
4. Behavior management pertaining to restraint or seclusion use.
5. Care or service provided to high-risk populations.
6. Needs, expectations, and satisfaction of individuals and organizations served.

Control charts may be used for displaying and tracking many—if not all—of the areas listed. For example, an *np* chart may be used to display the number of patients in restraints for a regular, given time frame. Another example involves the medication use measurement. There are various aspects of medication use (for instance, ordering, distributing, handling, therapeutic benefits, and adverse drug reactions). A *u* chart may be used to display the number of items handled correctly for patients regarding medication use in all of the categories previously listed.

The systematic collection of data will be enhanced by an operational definition and check sheet, as discussed previously in this book. The operational definition involves defining who will gather the data, what type of data are being gathered, and exactly how the data will be gathered. Data will also be systematically collected when the measurement activities are included in existing processes, rather than as separate activities. Flowcharts of key processes should contain rectangles (activities) that designate data gathering and diamonds (decisions) that illustrate actions taken within the process based on the results of the data collection.

Collecting and Comparing Data

4. The data from the measurements are collected over time and compared with current data from other sources.

   Within the data inventory, time frames are established for measurement of key processes. Many processes do not require 100 percent measurement. In these cases, the healthcare organization establishes the frequency of measurement and is evaluated by JCAHO on its ability to fulfill its measurement time schedule.

   Measurements for processes and outcomes designated by the healthcare organization should be compared with data from other organizations. This may be performed as a benchmarking activity when examining processes. Benchmarking generally involves the identification of an external organization, or internal department that performs the same process you do, but does it better than you. Rather than just comparing your numbers to their numbers, an effort is made to examine how the "best practices" organization performs the process. If the demographic factors allow transference of the process, it may be adopted by your organization.

There are many books available to assist healthcare organizations in benchmarking steps. There are also benchmarking partnerships available through various organizations. When embarking on benchmarking activities, take the time to research ways to get the most from your activities. This includes doing preparatory work prior to the actual benchmarking endeavor such as flowcharting and gathering baseline data. It is critical that those individuals involved in benchmarking have an excellent understanding of their own processes before obtaining data about other organizations' processes.

The comparison-of-data requirement is also fulfilled by participation in a comparative database as now required by JCAHO. The healthcare organization must select appropriate clinical measures and enroll in an external database that has been approved by JCAHO. The healthcare organization sends data to the external database and receives quarterly comparative reports. If the organization's measurements are significantly worse than the others in the comparative database, the organization must evaluate the data and take action. The action taken will generally involve use of the PI tools and techniques and may result in new processes or redesign of existing processes.

Utilization of Statistical Methods

5. Statistical methods are utilized. Common and special cause variation are examined, and action is taken when appropriate.

   JCAHO surveyors are looking for active use of the tools and techniques as outlined in this book. In the past, organizations have often failed to respond to undesirable data trends. Even when they did occasionally respond, the result was generally a quick-fix approach that lacked a thoughtful determination of root causes. JCAHO's response to that has been to place an emphasis on statistical tools and data-driven decisions.

One of the biggest changes in the standards is the requirement that healthcare organizations identify common and special cause variation. By including a single sentence relating to common and special cause variability, JCAHO has effectively required that accredited healthcare organizations use control charts! This has been overlooked by many healthcare organizations because it has not been understood. Even some of the surveyors have had to learn what is intended by this standard. However, as time goes on, the use of control charts will dramatically increase in healthcare organizations.

Another JCAHO standard that relates to control chart use concerns process stability. JCAHO has several standards that require organizations to determine if their processes are stable. The way to do this is to place the data on a control chart, then evaluate the control chart using the rules given in chapter 3. When special cause is present, we say that the process is *out-of-control.* Another way to interpret this situation is to say that the process is *unstable.* A stable process does not have special cause variation. It exhibits only common cause variation and is in-control.

Redesign of Existing Processes and the Design of New Processes

6. A format is followed for the redesign of existing processes and the design of new processes. The format includes baseline performance expectations.

   The healthcare organization's PI Plan should outline the procedure for designing and redesigning processes. It is important that everyone involved in these activities throughout the organization follow this procedure. In addition, evidence should be maintained of these activities, such as copies of flowcharts and process data. A sample format for the redesign of processes follows. The steps for designing new processes are similar to the ones outlined.

Steps in the redesign of existing processes:

a. Form a team that includes representation from all areas affected by the process.

b. Appoint a facilitator, set meeting dates, timelines, and team objectives.

c. Flowchart the process.

d. Establish measurements within the process, including a baseline measurement.

e. Gather baseline measurement data.

f. If necessary, use a Pareto chart and Ishikawa Diagram to address problems in the existing process.

g. Benchmark the process by exploring how others perform the same process.

h. Establish performance expectations for the process based on customer feedback.

i. Flowchart the proposed redesigned process.

j. Pilot test the redesigned process if possible, if not do full-scale implementation.

k. Gather data from the redesigned process to compare to baseline data and performance expectations.

l. Evaluate the data and make a decision to adopt and standardize the process or continue to redesign the process.

m. Establish accountability for continuing to monitor the process and look for continued improvements.

n. Disband the team if the monitoring and continued improvements are outside the team or can be performed by individuals.

One of the PI standards relating to new and redesigned processes focuses on baseline measurements. In establishing baseline measurements, identify events that can detect changes in performance and allow for comparison over time. When choosing the item to be measured, it is important to concentrate on items that are important to the customer.

Conclusion

This overview of the PI standards as they relate to the tools and techniques in quality is intended as a supplement to bridge the QI tools with PI. Often, organizations attempt to fulfill the PI standards by creating a paper trail that has little or no day-to-day reality or benefit. Unfortunately, there is little to gain (besides possible accreditation) from playing the paper game. In this time of limited resources in which most healthcare organizations find themselves, it is imperative to make the standards provide a return on investment. Organizations can make the PI standards work for them by embracing the quality philosophy of continuous improvement while fulfilling JCAHO's PI standards.

EXERCISE

Answer the questions below to the best of your ability either individually or in a group discussion.

1. What organizations currently require that your healthcare institution gather data?
2. What kinds of data (that you are aware of) must be gathered for the organizations listed in question 1?
3. What kinds of data should you be gathering to evaluate the effectiveness of your organization toward your strategic objectives (according to your strategic plan)?
4. Are you aware of any duplicative data-gathering procedures, or any data gathering that may be discontinued? If so, please list/discuss.
5. If your organization were to distribute the data inventory form, who would it go to?

Reference

Ackoff, R. 1994. *The Democratic Corporation.* New York: Oxford University Press.

Answers to Exercises

ANSWERS TO CHAPTER 3 EXERCISES

Figure 3.11

a. This control chart is ❑ in control (go to next question)
☒ out-of-control (continue with this question)

b. Specifically, the problem with this chart is:
7 consecutive points below the center line

Figure 3.12

a. This control chart is ❑ in control (go to next question)
☒ out-of-control (continue with this question)

b. Specifically, the problem with this chart is:
7 consecutive increasing points

Figure 3.13

a. This control chart is ❑ in control (go to next question)
☒ out-of-control (continue with this question)

b. Specifically, the problem with this chart is:
4/5 points are hugging the center line

Figure 3.14

a. This control chart is ❑ in control (go to next question)
☒ out-of-control (continue with this question)

b. Specifically, the problem with this chart is:
a cyclical pattern

Figure 3.15

a. This control chart is ☒ in control (go to next question)

Figure 3.16

a. This control chart is ❑ in control (go to next question)
☒ out-of-control (continue with this question)

b. Specifically, the problem with this chart is:
there are two points outside of the upper control limit

ANSWERS TO EXERCISE 4.1

CHART

__A__ 1. Number of delinquent medical record charts.

__A__ 2. Daily patient census (number of patients in the hospital).

__V__ 3. Patient accounts receivable balances.

__V__ 4. Patient cholesterol levels.

__V__ 5. Average length of stay.

__V__ 6. Scheduled appointment time less time at which patient arrived.

__A__ 7. Completed history and physicals (H&P) on the chart.

__A__ 8. Patient satisfied or not.

__V__ 9. Patient satisfaction level on a 1–5 scale.

__V__ 10. Average age of patients on a unit.

__V__ 11. Average salary level for hospital nursing staff.

__A__ 12. Percent of patients with third-party insurance.

__V__ 13. Time that patients wait before seeing a physician.

ANSWERS TO EXERCISE 4.2

CHART

Chart	
np	1. The number of post-operative major discrepancies recorded by month.
$\bar{X}$ and *s*	2. The average satisfaction level (from 1–5) from a patient survey given monthly to 25 patients chosen randomly.
p	3. The percent of job interviewees who fail to keep their appointments.
Indiv/mr	4. The time it takes to do a certain patient procedure that occurs rarely, and is measured each time it occurs.
c	5. The number of repairs per unit for hospital equipment.
$\bar{X}$ and *R*	6. The average amount of time a sample of five Registered Nurses spend on administrative tasks.
np	7. The number of incident reports each month.
u	8. A 5 percent sample of employee records that are reviewed each month for four specific factors: evaluation done on time, credentials current, emergency forms in file, and training log up-to-date.
Indiv/mr	9. The time it takes to connect IV lines, recorded by individual patients.
$\bar{X}$ and *s*	10. A sample of 20 records per month to determine preadmission paperwork processing time.

ANSWERS TO CHAPTER 5 EXERCISES

STEP 1:

$$\bar{p} = \frac{27}{200} = 0.1350$$

STEP 2:

Upper control limit (UCL):

$$UCL p = 0.1350 + 3\sqrt{\frac{0.1350(1 - 0.1350)}{10}} = 0.4592$$

Lower control limit (LCL):

$$LCL p = 0.1350 - 3\sqrt{\frac{0.1350(1 - 0.1350)}{10}} = -0.1892 \text{ or } 0$$

STEP 3:

Figure 5.5 shows that there is one point outside of the upper control limit.

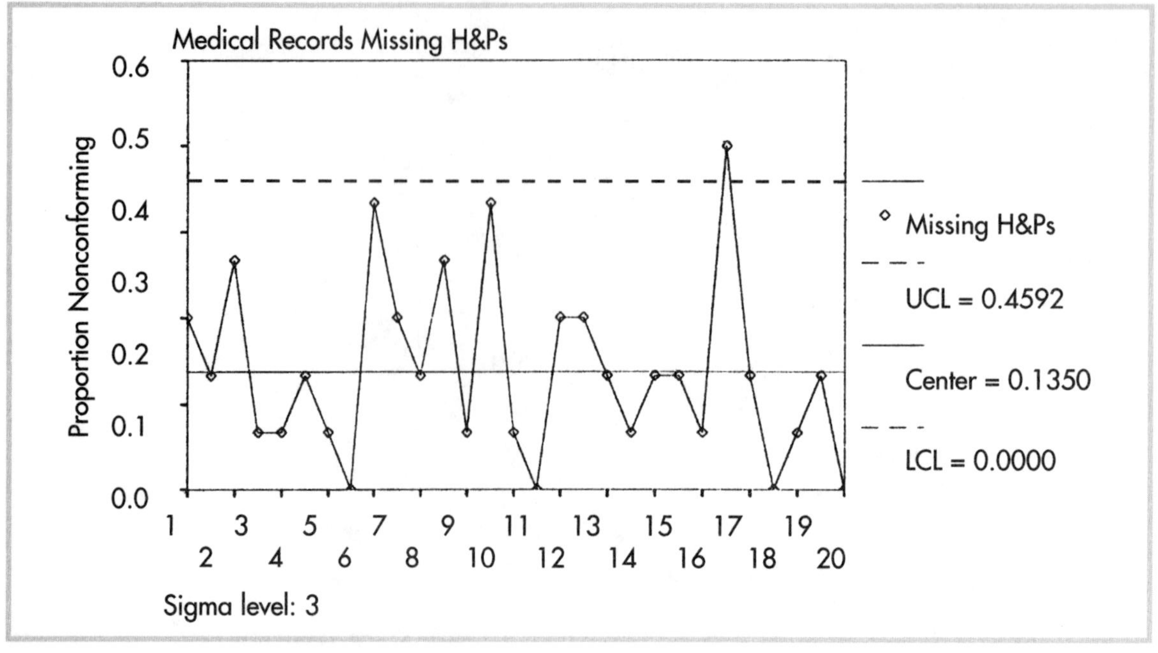

Figure 5.5. *p* chart.

ANSWERS TO CHAPTER 6 EXERCISES

The completed table is shown in Table 6.8.

Table 6.8.

Week	**1**	**2**	**3**	**4**	**5**	**6**	**7**	**8**	**9**	**10**
Test 1	15	24	5	12	35	10	25	15	15	32
Test 2	5	23	15	42	10	20	45	19	12	18
Test 3	35	30	25	28	24	15	30	23	29	10
Test 4	21	15	33	10	19	25	15	41	20	35
Test 5	23	10	34	26	20	25	34	38	10	42
Sum	99	102	112	118	108	95	149	136	86	137
Mean	19.8	20.4	22.4	23.6	21.6	19.0	29.8	27.2	17.2	27.4
Range	30	20	29	32	25	15	30	26	19	32

Week	**11**	**12**	**13**	**14**	**15**	**16**	**17**	**18**	**19**	**20**
Test 1	14	13	25	31	18	45	14	26	36	22
Test 2	12	32	12	42	20	25	23	42	11	3
Test 3	31	34	26	28	12	13	18	19	39	31
Test 4	30	15	13	12	25	18	25	28	24	20
Test 5	24	25	18	17	32	35	29	35	22	5
Sum	111	119	94	130	107	136	109	150	132	81
Mean	22.2	23.8	18.8	26.0	21.4	27.2	21.8	30.0	26.4	16.2
Range	19	21	14	30	20	32	15	23	28	28

Step 1: Complete Table 6.8 to assist in calculating the center lines for the $\bar{X}$ and R charts:

Center line (CL):

$$\bar{\bar{X}} = \frac{462.20}{20} = 23.11$$

$$\bar{R} = \frac{488}{20} = 24.40$$

Step 2: Calculate UCL and LCL for the $\bar{X}$ chart:

Upper control limit (UCL) $\bar{X}$ chart:

$$\text{UCL}\bar{X} = 23.11 + (0.577 \times 24.40) = 37.18$$

Lower control limit (LCL) $\bar{X}$ chart:

$$\text{LCL}\bar{X} = 23.11 - (0.577 \times 24.40) = 9.03$$

Step 3: Calculate UCL and LCL for the R chart:

Upper control limit (UCL) R Chart:

$$\text{UCL}R = 2.114 \times 24.40 = 51.58$$

Lower control limit (LCL) R chart:

$$\text{LCL}R = 0 \times 24.40 = 0$$

Step 4: Draw the control chart.

As mentioned earlier, when performing calculations by hand versus calculations on the computer, there is often a slight discrepancy between the two in the numbers below the decimal point. This is because of rounding error. In these situations, the computer-generated control chart is considered the more accurate.

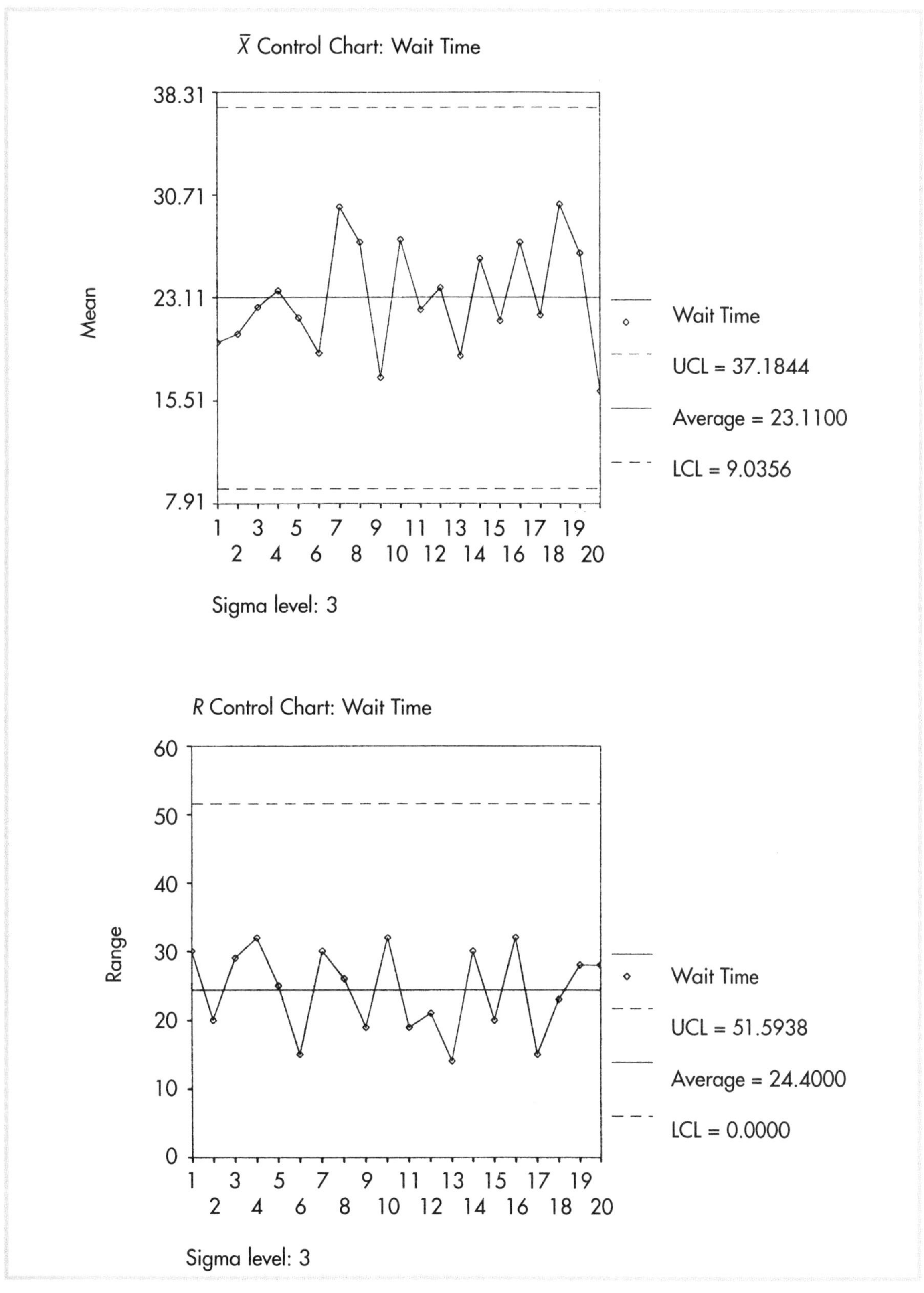

Figure 6.4. $\bar{X}$ and *R* control charts.

ANSWERS TO EXERCISE 8.1

Complete the grid below by placing the appropriate tool in the box on the right. You may use some tools more than once.

What You Want to Do:	Tool You Will Use:
Find out to what degree things are causing a particular problem.	Pareto chart
Gather data in an efficient manner.	Check sheet
Determine possible root causes of a problem.	Ishikawa Diagram
Understand the steps involved in a process.	Process flowchart
Learn what others are doing in the field regarding a specified process.	Benchmarking
Standardize a change in the process.	Process flowchart
Monitor data over time.	Control chart
Help ensure the data are gathered by everyone in the same manner.	Operational definition
Help lead a group discussion to determine inputs into a problem.	Ishikawa Diagram
Display the inputs in problems in a manner that makes it clear which ones are the biggest causes of the problem.	Pareto chart
See if the change you made to the process has improved the process.	Control chart

Index